Gasdynamic Lasers: An Introduction

QUANTUM ELECTRONICS — PRINCIPLES AND APPLICATIONS

A Series of Monographs

EDITED BY

YOH-HAN PAO
Case Western Reserve University
Cleveland, Ohio

N. S. Kapany and J. J. Burke. Optical Waveguides, 1972

Dietrich Marcuse. Theory of Dielectric Optical Waveguides, 1974

Benjamin Chu. Laser Light Scattering, 1974

Bruno Crosignani, Paolo Di Porto, and Mario Bertolotti. Statistical Properties of Scattered Light, 1975

John D. Anderson, Jr. Gasdynamic Lasers: An Introduction, 1976

In preparation

W. W. Duley. CO_2 Lasers: Effects and Applications

Gasdynamic Lasers: An Introduction

JOHN D. ANDERSON, JR.

Department of Aerospace Engineering
University of Maryland
College Park, Maryland

ACADEMIC PRESS New York San Francisco London 1976

A Subsidiary of Harcourt Brace Jovanovich, Publishers

ACADEMIC PRESS, INC.
111 Fifth Avenue, New York, New York 10003

United Kingdom Edition published by
ACADEMIC PRESS, INC. (LONDON) LTD.
24/28 Oval Road, London NW1

Library of Congress Cataloging in Publication Data

Anderson, John David.
Gasdynamic lasers.

(Quantum electronics series)
Bibliography: p.
Includes index.
1. Gas lasers. I. Title.
TA1695.A5 621.36'63 75-16875
ISBN 0-12-056950-7

PRINTED IN THE UNITED STATES OF AMERICA

Contents

Preface

Lasers (light amplification by stimulated emission of radiation) have been part of modern science and technology for only a short fifteen years; yet during that time they have experienced a rate of growth and achieved a maturity that have been almost phenomenal in the history of physical science. In addition, the applications of the monochromatic, highly columnated visible or infrared beams of radiation produced by these lasers have also multiplied at an equally phenomenal rate. It is safe to say that the laser has become a permanent fixture in most modern physics, chemistry, and engineering laboratories. Moreover, even the layman is generally acquainted with the typical "garden variety" of low power lasers (such as the ruby or He–Ne lasers) from science classes, technology museums, demonstrations, or direct professional use.

This book does not deal with typical "garden variety" lasers. Instead, it focuses on the gasdynamic laser—a revolutionary device which, in 1966, created a breakthrough in high energy laser technology. With the gasdynamic laser, the dream of producing laser beams transmitting tens or hundreds of kilowatts for durations of seconds, or even minutes, suddenly became a reality. To date, the gasdynamic laser has seen at least two major development generations, and its technology has matured to the state at which it can logically be presented in a text, studied, and analyzed. This is precisely the purpose of this book.

It is written for at least three groups of people: (1) students who are interested in studying an example of interdisciplinary applied science in action, (2) professional scientists and engineers who, without previous experience in this area, want to learn how and why gasdynamic lasers work, and (3) workers in the field who want a convenient review and reference source reflecting the fruits of their labor. In addition, gasdynamic laser technology overlaps the various fields of aerodynamics, physical chemistry, quantum mechanics, spectroscopy, and physical optics. The reader is *not* expected to be an expert in any or all of these fields. For this reason, the fundamental elements of each field are developed as needed for application to gasdynamic lasers. The intent is to provide a book from which readers with various backgrounds can obtain a coherent education in gasdynamic lasers.

The style of the book is intentionally informal. The author sees no reason for a technical or scientific text to be rigid or sterile in its presentation; instead, the present book attempts to "talk" to the reader, hopefully guiding him along the paths from fundamental principles to specific applications with a minimum of confusion and a maximum of interest. The science and technology associated with gasdynamic lasers is exciting and challenging. The intent here is to convey this excitement and to give the reader the extent of pleasure that should go hand-in-hand with the acquisition of new knowledge.

Acknowledgments

Through the kindness of Dr. Kurt Enkenhus of the Naval Ordnance Laboratory and Dr. John Wendt of the von Karman Institute, the author was invited to give the lectures on gasdynamic lasers during a course on "High Power Gas Lasers" presented at the von Karman Institute for Fluid Dynamics, Brussels, Belgium, in March 1974. During and after this course, numerous students approached the author, suggesting that the lectures be amplified into a book on gasdynamic lasers. Their encouragement was so compelling and emphatic that it could not be ignored. This book, considerably extended and amplified in depth and scope over the original lectures, is the result.

Some other acknowledgments are due. First, the state-of-the-art of gasdynamic lasers exemplified by this book was developed through the toil, efforts, insight, and intelligence of numerous teams of engineers and scientists in laboratories throughout industry, government, and universities. It is impractical to list them all here, but their work is detailed throughout this book. The author wishes to give special acknowledgment to his colleagues of seven years at the Naval Ordnance Laboratory, especially John Vamos and Mike Plummer, who obtained considerable gasdynamic laser data from experiments with a shock tube; Richard Humphrey and Eva Winkler, who converted an arc tunnel to a gasdynamic laser; Walter Glowacki, Michael Madden, and Jerry Wagner, who performed various analyses; and E. Leroy Harris, who guided all of us in the right direction. The author is proud to be listed among these ranks.

There is one other ingredient in all books of this nature, and that is the huge amount of time necessary to prepare the material in a fashion that can be digested by the reader. The author gives special thanks to his wife, Sarah-Allen, and his daughters, Katherine and Elizabeth, who relinquished hours upon hours of valuable family time with their husband and father so that he could accomplish this task. Also appreciated are the many hours of work spent by Mrs. Edna Brothers in typing the manuscript. To all of these friends and loved-ones, the author says thank you, and breathes a sigh of relief.

Chapter I

Introduction

High energy gas lasers are a modern reality. It is now feasible to produce near-diffraction-limited laser beams with cross-sectional areas the size of the cover of this book, transmitting hundreds of kilowatts for durations of seconds or minutes depending on the practical design and capacity of the gas supply and hardware components of the device. This statement could not have been made ten years ago. What has spearheaded this breakthrough in high energy laser devices in the past decade? The answer—gasdynamic lasers—is the subject of this book.

In 1965, the only high energy gas lasers operating on a practical basis were conventional electric discharge lasers [see Patel (1968) for a particularly lucid description of the CO_2 electric discharge laser]. In such devices the laser gas is produced by an electric discharge that not only ionizes the gas to sustain the discharge itself, but that also preferentially excites various vibrational or electronic energy levels of the molecules or atoms. Such preferential excitation can result in a population inversion; hence laser action occurs. It is commonplace to obtain watts, and even a few kilowatts, of continuous wave power from such lasers. However, conventional electric discharge lasers are not easily scaled to arbitrarily large sizes and powers because the physics of electric discharges favors undesirable arcing in large scale devices, and the heating of the laser gas by the discharge can reduce or even destroy the population inversion, hence terminating the laser action. This latter objection can be partly overcome by flowing the gas at high speeds (subsonic or even supersonic) through the laser cavity. Nevertheless, in 1965, hopes for a truly high power gas laser were languishing; the best that could be obtained was about 9 kW from laser tubes about 200 ft long!

However, the seeds for a revolution in high power gas lasers were planted in 1962 by Basov and Oraevskii (1963), who suggested that population inversions in molecular systems could be created by rapid heating or cooling of the system. Subsequently, Hurle and Hertzberg (1965) suggested that such cooling and population inversions could be obtained in the rapid, nonequilibrium expansion of an initially hot gas through a supersonic nozzle. They considered the specific case of electronic level inversions in expanding Xe but were unsuccessful in measuring such inversions in the laboratory. Then, Kantrowitz (1946) combined this idea with his previous work on vibrational nonequilibrium in CO_2, and, in 1966, he and a group of physicists and engineers at the Avco Everett Research Laboratory operated the first gasdynamic laser, using a mixture of CO_2–N_2–H_2O (see Gerry, 1970).

These events were truly revolutionary. To fully appreciate this, first consider in your imagination a supersonic wind tunnel such as those commonly found in many aerodynamic laboratories. However, when this particular tunnel is turned on, we do *not* measure the lift and drag on an aerodynamic model or the pressure and heat transfer distributions over a surface. Instead, when the switch is thrown for this particular tunnel, we see *a very powerful laser beam propagating from the test section.* Indeed, this is not a wind tunnel at all, but rather it is a *gasdynamic laser.*

As shown schematically in Fig. 1.1, a gasdynamic laser takes a hot, high pressure mixture of gases (usually CO_2, N_2, and H_2O or He) and expands this mixture very rapidly through a supersonic nozzle. During the expansion, the gas is turned into a laser medium (i.e., a population inversion is created). The supersonic laser gas then passes into the test

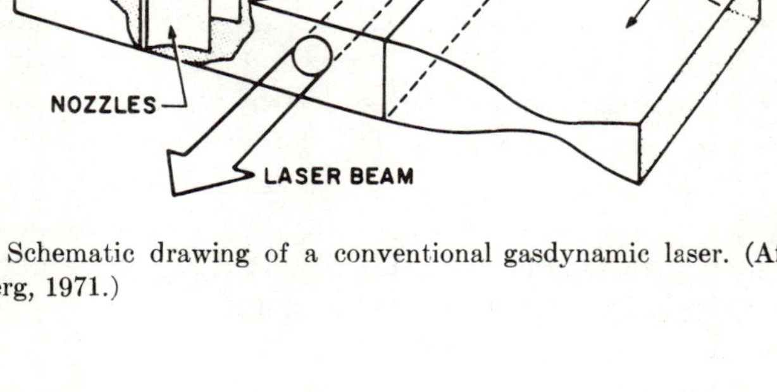

FIG. 1.1 Schematic drawing of a conventional gasdynamic laser. (After Monsler and Greenberg, 1971.)

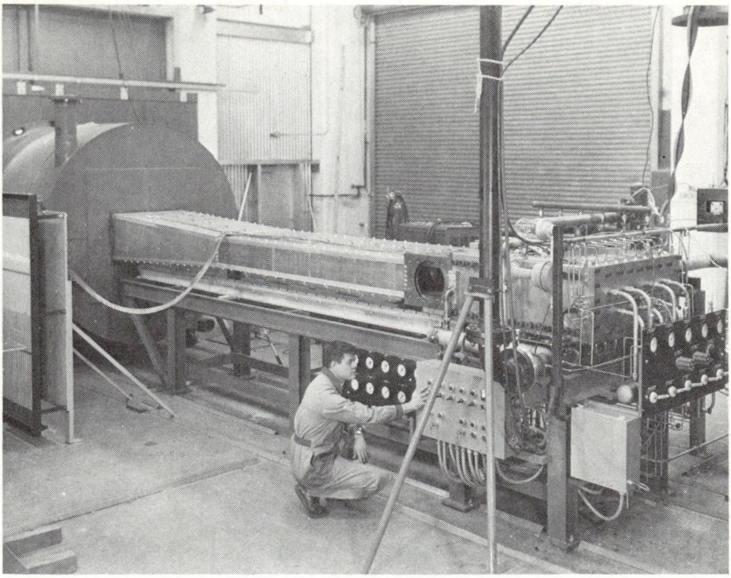

FIG. 1.2 135 kW gasdynamic laser at Avco Everett Research Laboratory, Inc. (After Gerry, 1970.)

section (laser cavity) where, if mirrors are placed on both sides of the test section, a beam of laser energy is extracted perpendicular to the flow. The supersonic stream then enters a diffuser where it is shocked down to subsonic speeds and generally exhausted to the atmosphere.

The revolutionary aspect of a gasdynamic laser is that, unlike the early electric discharge lasers with their attendant problems of arc discharges in large volumes, gasdynamic lasers can be scaled to large sizes without major physical complications. This is because the population inversions are produced by purely thermal means within the supersonic expansion, and such gasdynamic processes are not dependent on the lateral extent of the supersonic flow. For example, a multimode, continuous wave power output of 60 kW from a CO_2–N_2–H_2O gasdynamic laser has been reported by Gerry (1970), and an average laser power of 400 kW has been extracted for 4 msec from a shock tube gasdynamic laser by Klosterman and Hoffman (1973) working in the laser group at the University of Washington. A picture of a large-scale gasdynamic laser is shown in Fig. 1.2.

As part of the early development of the gasdynamic laser, Basov *et al.* (1968) carried out a theoretical analysis of population inversions in CO_2–N_2 expanding mixtures and predicted that substantial inversions can indeed occur under suitable conditions for the gas mixture ratio and the nozzle reservoir pressure and temperature. However, Basov missed an essential point, namely, that the inclusion of a "catalyst" such as H_2O or He is necessary for the attainment of reasonable population inversions. Basov used older values of the vibrational energy exchange rates, which resulted in optimistic values of the population inversions; indeed, using more recent rates as compiled by Taylor and Bitterman (1969), Anderson (1970c) has shown that the CO_2–N_2 mixtures considered by Basov *et al.* do not yield significant inversions. The group at Avco first recognized this fact and have reported experiments using CO_2–N_2–H_2O mixtures as early as 1966. Theoretical calculations showing the beneficial role of H_2O were reported by Anderson (1970c) in 1969. The exact role of H_2O or He as a catalyst is discussed later in this book.

Since these initial experiments and calculations, the technology and fundamental understanding of CO_2–N_2 gasdynamic lasers has grown precociously. This growth is exemplified by experiments carried out in arc tunnels (Lee and Gowen, 1971; Lee *et al.*, 1972; Anderson *et al.*, 1971b; Anderson and Winkler, 1971), shock tunnels (Klosterman and Hoffman, 1973; Anderson *et al.*, 1971b; Christiansen and Tsongas, 1971; Hertzberg *et al.*, 1972; Vamos, 1974; Tennant *et al.*, 1974; Kuehn and Monson, 1970), and combustion driven devices (Gerry, 1970; Tulip and Sequin, 1971; Yatsiv *et al.*, 1971; Meinzer, 1972), and by theoretical calculations reported by Basov *et al.* (1968), Anderson (1970c), Anderson *et al.* (1971b), Anderson and Winkler (1971), Anderson and Harris (1972a,b), Anderson (1972a,b, 1973, 1974), Hoffman and Vlases (1972), and Murty (1974). Moreover, gasdynamic lasers using CO as the lasing medium have also been demonstrated (McKenzie, 1972). It is the purpose of this book to bring the reader up-to-date in this exciting state-of-the-art, while at the same time developing the underlying physical and gasdynamic fundamentals that govern such devices.

Chapter II

Elementary Physics

Gasdynamic lasers are truly interdisciplinary devices. The concepts and design of gasdynamic lasers cut across such disciplines as quantum mechanics, statistical thermodynamics, physical chemistry, nonequilibrium gasdynamics, physical optics, and the aerodynamics of internal flows. It is unrealistic to assume that any single person is a master of all these fields; hence, wherever appropriate throughout this book, the fundamental physical principles underlying various aspects of gasdynamic lasers will be discussed in a somewhat self-contained manner. In particular, Chapters II, III, and IV discuss the basic detailed physical phenomena that ultimately are responsible for producing gasdynamic laser action. Comprehensive treatments of the background laser physics can be found in such books as Siegman (1971) and Lengyel (1971), and the fundamentals of nonequilibrium gasdynamics are thoroughly treated in Vincenti and Kruger (1965) and in Clarke and McChesney (1964). The necessary elements of quantum mechanics and statistical thermodynamics are nicely developed by Davidson (1962).

2.1 Energy Levels and Population Inversion

Consider a collection of molecules in a gas. Pick one of the molecules and examine it. The molecule is moving about in space—it has translational energy; it is rotating about its principal axes—hence it has rotational kinetic energy; the atoms that make up the molecule may be vibrating back and forth from some equilibrium position—it has vibrational kinetic and potential energy; and, finally, the electrons move about the nuclei of the molecule—hence it has kinetic and potential energy of electronic origin. However, the amazing quality of these various forms of molecular energy is that they *cannot* be any arbitrary value. Rather, one of the most important discoveries of modern physics is that the molecule, at any given instant, *has to occupy one of a very specific set of energy levels*; i.e., the energy values of a molecule are *quantized*. This is shown schematically in Fig. 2.1. Instead of one molecule, imagine the whole collection, say 10^6 molecules, and look at the first quantized energy level ϵ_0 (the ground state). There may be 400,000 molecules in this level at some instant in time. The number 400,000 is called the population N_0 of the ϵ_0 level. Next, look at the first excited level, ϵ_1; there may be 200,000 molecules in this level, hence $N_1 =$ 200,000 = the *population* of the ϵ_1 level, and so forth. The *set* of numbers, $N_0, N_1, N_2, \ldots, N_i, \ldots$ is called the *population distribution* over the energy levels of the gas. The *nature* of this population distribution is of vital importance for laser action. For example, consider the *vibrational energy* of a molecular gas. If the gas is in thermodynamic equilibrium, the population distribution will exponentially decrease with increasing ϵ_i, as shown in Fig. 2.2a; i.e., it will follow a Boltzmann distribution. A major characteristic of this equilibrium distribution is that $N_{i+1} < N_i$. However, if the gas is disturbed at any instant, say by means of an electric discharge or by a very sudden temperature change, then the population distribution can become a nonequilibrium distribution, and it is even possible that, at some instant, $N_{i+1} > N_i$. This situation, in which the number of molecules in a *higher* lying energy level is *greater* than the number in a *lower* lying level, is called a *population inversion*. The population inversion is the

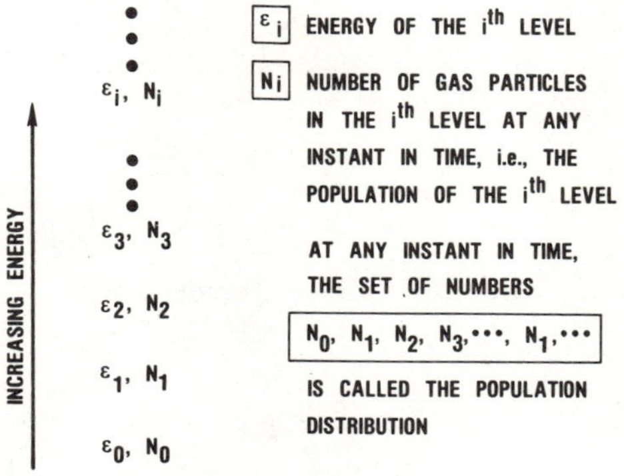

FIG. 2.1 Energy levels, populations, and population distributions.

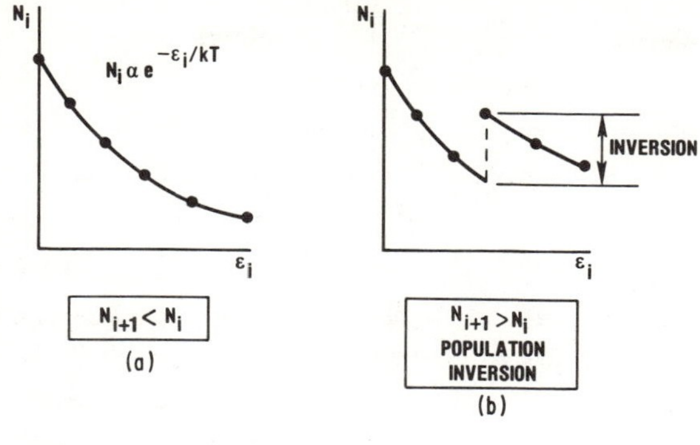

FIG. 2.2 (a) Equilibrium and (b) nonequilibrium vibrational population distributions; definition of population inversion.

essence of laser action, and the attainment of this population inversion by means of rapid cooling of the gas is the essence of a gasdynamic laser. Specifically, when a gas expands through a supersonic nozzle, as shown in Fig. 2.3, the gas temperature decreases very rapidly. Indeed, a fluid element moving through the nozzle can experience temperature changes as high as 10^6 degrees/sec in the throat region of the nozzle. In fact, expansion through a minimum-length supersonic nozzle is the fastest practical means of cooling a gas. Therefore, it is reasonable to expect that, for certain conditions, a population inversion can be created in such an expansion.

With the above discussion in mind, the pivotal and first problem in studying, understanding, and analyzing a gasdynamic laser is to examine the *nonequilibrium flow through a nozzle* and the behavior of this flow as it moves downstream through the laser cavity. Specifically, we wish to calculate the population distribution as it varies through the nozzle for a mixture of CO_2–N_2 and H_2O or He, and we wish to examine the conditions under which a population inversion will develop. This will be the subject

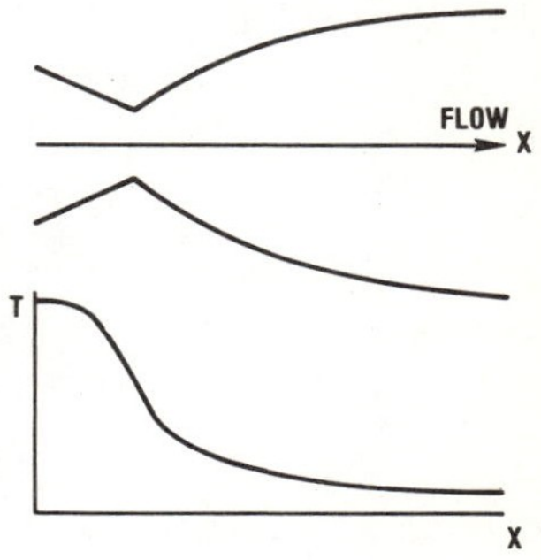

FIG. 2.3 Static temperature variation through a convergent-divergent supersonic nozzle.

of Chapter IV. However, before we address this problem, we should answer the following question.

2.2 Why Does a Population Inversion Make a Laser Work?

Consider two energy levels of the molecules in a gas. There are three mechanisms by which these energy levels interact with radiation: spontaneous emission, stimulated emission, and absorption. These are illustrated in Fig. 2.4.

Now, consider a single molecule in a field of radiation where the radiative intensity per unit frequency is I_ν.

$(A_{21})_\nu \equiv$ number of spontaneous radiative transitions per second per particle per unit frequency. This is called the Einstein spontaneous emission coefficient, and sometimes the Einstein transition probability.

$(B_{21})_\nu I_\nu \equiv$ number of induced radiative transitions per second per particle per unit frequency. $(B_{21})_\nu$ is the Einstein induced emission coefficient.

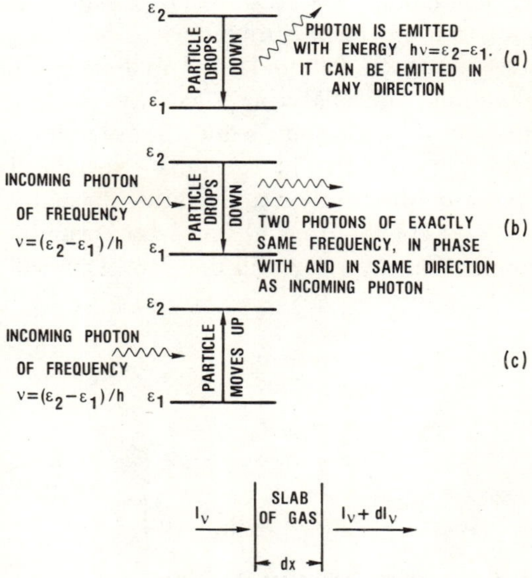

FIG. 2.4 Schematic of the radiative processes of (a) spontaneous and (b) stimulated emission and (c) absorption.

$(B_{12})_\nu I_\nu \equiv$ number of radiative transitions per second per particle per unit frequency due to absorption. $(B_{12})_\nu$ is the Einstein absorption coefficient.

Consider a slab of gas of geometric thickness dx, as shown in Fig. 2.4. Let I_ν be the radiative intensity (energy per second per unit area) incident on the left side of the slab, and let $(dI)_\nu$ be the change in intensity while traversing the slab. Also, let N_1 and N_2 be the number of molecules per unit volume in the ϵ_1 and ϵ_2 energy levels, respectively. Then, from the above definitions, we can simply write down

$$(dI)_\nu = [\underbrace{(A_{21})_\nu N_2}_{\substack{\text{spontaneous}\\ \text{emission}}} + \underbrace{(B_{21})_\nu I_\nu N_2}_{\substack{\text{induced}\\ \text{emission}}} - \underbrace{(B_{12})_\nu I_\nu N_1}_{\text{absorption}}]h\nu\, dx \tag{2.1}$$

For the infrared wavelengths characteristic of molecular lasers, the spontaneous emission is negligible. Also, in general, $(B_{21})_\nu = (g_1/g_2)(B_{12})_\nu$, as shown by Anderson and Winkler (1971) and in most modern physics textbooks. Here, g_1 and g_2 are statistical weights of the levels. Hence, Eq. (2.1) becomes

$$\frac{(dI)_\nu}{I_\nu} = (B_{12})_\nu \left(\frac{g_1}{g_2} N_2 - N_1\right) h\nu\, dx \tag{2.2}$$

Now we can answer our original question. Looking at Eq. (2.2), $(dI)_\nu/I_\nu$ will be positive when $[(g_1/g_2)N_2 - N_1] > 0$, i.e., when a population inversion exists between the ϵ_2 and ϵ_1 energy levels. Hence, a *population inversion leads to an amplification of the radiative intensity* I_ν. This is the laser effect, and this is why a population inversion makes a laser work!

2.3 Definition and Calculation of Small-Signal Gain

The small-signal laser gain is an extremely important figure of merit for gas laser devices; it is to laser physicists what lift and drag coefficients are to aerodynamicists. It is also a direct measurement of the population inversion. Everything else being equal, the higher the small-signal gain the easier laser action can be obtained in a gas. Therefore, because we have just discussed the reasons why a population inversion makes a laser work, we now extend this discussion to the analysis of small-signal gain. Also, the following results are necessary for our subsequent discussions on the theory and experimental measurements of gasdynamic laser performance.

Let us consider stimulated emission and absorption, ignoring spontaneous emission as stated previously. Consider again the slab of gas of geometric thickness dx with radiation of intensity I_ν (per unit frequency) incident normally on the slab as shown in Fig. 2.4. The radiative intensity absorbed *in a given spectral line* of the gas is $(dI)_\nu$ (per unit frequency). Due to line broadening effects in the gas (natural, Doppler, and collision), $(dI)_\nu$ varies over a narrow frequency range, as shown in Fig. 2.5. This gives rise to the *line shape*. The intensity of radiation between ν and $\nu + d\nu$ is $(dI)_\nu\, d\nu$. The integrated radiative intensity (total intensity absorbed by the line) is

$$dI = \int_\nu (dI)_\nu\, d\nu$$

The spectral absorption coefficient α_ν is *defined* as

$$(dI)_\nu = -\alpha_\nu I_\nu\, dx \tag{2.3}$$

Examining Eq. (2.3), if I_ν *decreases* as it traverses the slab of gas, then dI_ν is negative and α_ν is a positive number. On the other hand, if I_ν increases as in the laser effect, then dI_ν is positive and α_ν has to be a negative quantity. Rather than deal with a "negative absorption coefficient," we define a new coefficient as

$$(dI)_\nu = G_{0_\nu} I_\nu\, dx \tag{2.4}$$

where G_0 is the *small-signal gain coefficient.*

$$G_{0_\nu} = -\alpha_\nu \tag{2.5}$$

Since the small-signal gain coefficient is the same as a "negative absorption coefficient," let us pursue our discussion in terms of the absorption coefficient. Comparing Eqs. (2.2) and (2.3), we see that

$$\alpha_\nu = h\nu (B_{12})_\nu \left(N_1 - \frac{g_1}{g_2} N_2 \right) \tag{2.6}$$

It is common to express $(B_{12})_\nu$ in terms of the Einstein coefficient for spontaneous emission $(A_{21})_\nu$, where (see, for example, Lengyel, 1971)

$$(A_{21})_\nu = \frac{8\pi h\nu^3}{c^2} (B_{12})_\nu$$

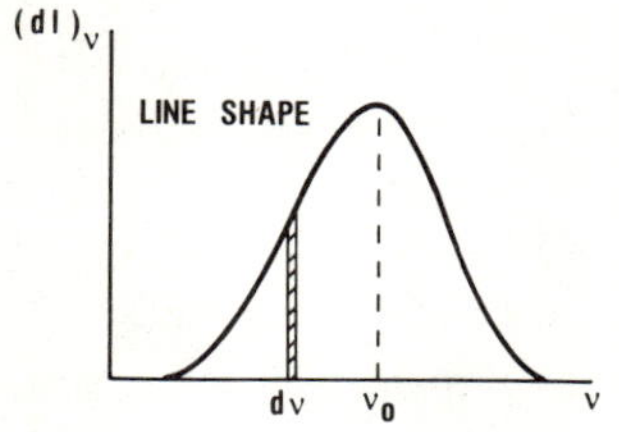

FIG. 2.5 Line shape of a spectral line.

Thus, Eq. (2.6) becomes

$$\alpha_\nu = \frac{c^2}{8\pi\nu^2} (A_{21})_\nu \left(N_1 - \frac{g_1}{g_2} N_2 \right) \tag{2.7}$$

Equation (2.7) gives the *spectral* absorption coefficient α_ν. Define the *integrated* absorption coefficient as $\int \alpha_\nu \, d\nu$, where the integral is taken over the entire spectral line.

Thus

$$\int_\nu \alpha_\nu \, d\nu = \frac{c^2}{8\pi\nu^2} \left(N_1 - \frac{g_1}{g_2} N_2 \right) \int_\nu (A_{21})_\nu \, d\nu \tag{2.8}$$

Note: The interval of integration over ν is small (lines are usually narrow), so that ν in the factor $c^2/8\pi\nu^2$ in Eq. (2.8) can be considered constant. Letting $\int (A_{21})_\nu \, d\nu \equiv A_{21}$, we have

$$\int_\nu \alpha_\nu \, d\nu = \frac{c^2}{8\pi\nu^2} A_{21} \left(N_1 - \frac{g_1}{g_2} N_2 \right) \tag{2.9}$$

Since $c/\nu = \lambda$, Eq. (2.9) becomes

$$\int_\nu \alpha_\nu \, d\nu = \frac{\lambda^2}{8\pi} A_{21} \left(N_1 - \frac{g_1}{g_2} N_2 \right) \tag{2.10}$$

Equation (2.10) gives the *integrated* absorption coefficient. Equation (2.10) is more useful than Eq. (2.7) because A_{21}, *not* $(A_{21})_\nu$, is available from laboratory measurements. To see this more clearly, recall Eq. (2.2).

$$(dI)_\nu = -(B_{12})_\nu \left(N_1 - \frac{g_1}{g_2} N_2 \right) I_\nu h\nu \, dx$$

$$(dI)_\nu = \frac{c^2}{8\pi h\nu^3} (A_{21})_\nu \left(N_1 - \frac{g_1}{g_2} N_2 \right) I_\nu h\nu \, dx$$

$$(dI)_\nu = \frac{\lambda^2}{8\pi} (A_{21})_\nu \left(N_1 - \frac{g_1}{g_2} N_2 \right) I_\nu \, dx \tag{2.11}$$

Now, integrate Eq. (2.11) over the thickness of the slab. Let L be the slab thickness

$$\int_{I_{\nu\text{in}}}^{I_{\nu\text{out}}} \frac{(dI)_\nu}{I_\nu} = -\frac{\lambda^2}{8\pi} (A_{21})_\nu \left(N_1 - \frac{g_1}{g_2} N_2 \right) \int_0^L dx$$

$$\frac{I_{\nu_{\text{out}}}}{I_{\nu_{\text{in}}}} = \exp\left(-\frac{\lambda^2}{8\pi} (A_{21})_\nu \left(N_1 - \frac{g_1}{g_2} N_2 \right) L \right)$$

For small values of the exponent, i.e., small L,

$$\frac{I_{\nu_{\text{out}}}}{I_{\nu_{\text{in}}}} = 1 - \frac{\lambda^2}{8\pi}(A_{21})_\nu\left(N_1 - \frac{g_1}{g_2}N_2\right)L + \cdots \tag{2.12}$$

The total radiative intensity *absorbed* over the *entire* spectral line is I_{abs}, where

$$I_{\text{abs}} \equiv \int_\nu (I_{\nu_{\text{in}}} - I_{\nu_{\text{out}}})\, d\nu \tag{2.13}$$

Assume that a continuous light source is used in an absorption experiment; i.e., $I_{\nu_{\text{in}}}$ is constant over the frequency interval of the spectral line. Combining Eqs. (2.12) and (2.13):

$$I_{\text{abs}} = \int_\nu \left[I_{\nu_{\text{in}}} - I_{\nu_{\text{in}}} + I_{\nu_{\text{in}}}\frac{\lambda^2}{8\pi}(A_{21})_\nu\left(N_1 - \frac{g_1}{g_2}N_2\right)L\right] d\nu$$

$$I_{\text{abs}} = I_{\nu_{\text{in}}}\frac{\lambda^2}{8\pi}\left(N_1 - \frac{g_1}{g_2}N_2\right)L\int_\nu (A_{21})_\nu\, d\nu$$

$$I_{\text{abs}} = \frac{\lambda^2 A_{21}}{8\pi}\left(N_1 - \frac{g_1}{g_2}N_2\right)LI_{\nu_{\text{in}}} \tag{2.14}$$

I_{abs} is *measured* in the lab. In turn, A_{21} is calculated from Eq. (2.14). Therefore, it is A_{21}, *not* $(A_{21})_\nu$, that is usually obtained from experiment. Thus, as stated earlier, Eq. (2.10) for the *integrated* absorption coefficient is more directly related to experimental observation than is Eq. (2.7) for the *spectral* absorption coefficient. Also, keep in mind that A_{21} is a *physical constant* of the molecule.

We have seen that in a conventional absorption experiment using a continuous light source, it is the *integrated* absorption coefficient $\int \alpha_\nu\, d\nu$, and hence A_{21}, that is obtained from the data. Values for A_{21}, and also for

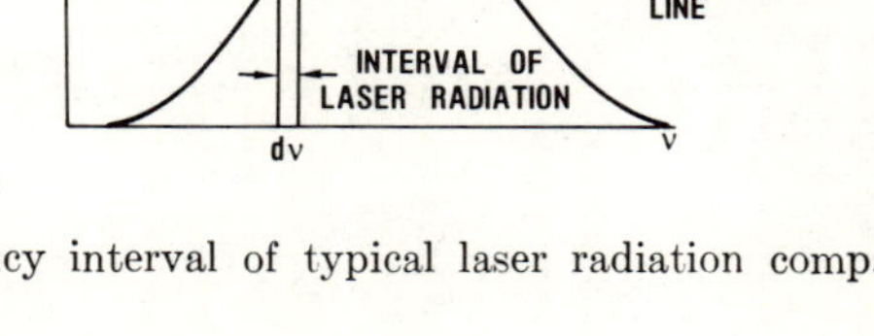

FIG. 2.6 Frequency interval of typical laser radiation compared with a typical spectral line shape.

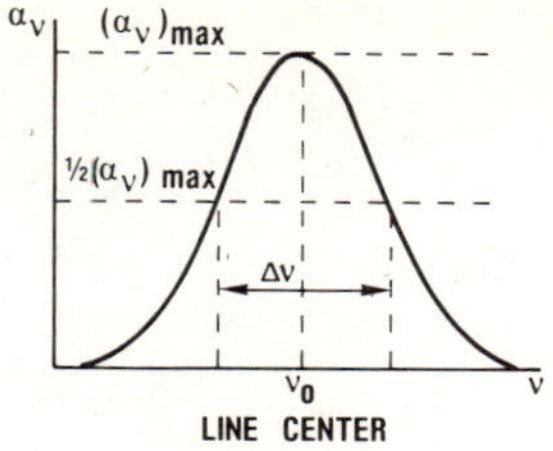

FIG. 2.7 Definition of line width for a spectral line.

the radiative lifetime,

$$\tau \equiv 1/A_{21}$$

are commonly quoted in the literature.

Now, consider *laser radiation*. This radiation is highly monochromatic. The laser cavity is generally tuned to emit radiation over a very small frequency interval. This interval is usually much smaller than the line width of a spectral line, as shown in Fig. 2.6. Hence, the absorption coefficient measured with *laser* radiation is the *spectral* absorption coefficient α_ν.

Now, let us relate α_ν to the integrated absorption coefficient and to A_{21}. Define a line shape *factor* $g(\nu, \nu_0)$ as

$$\alpha_\nu = g(\nu, \nu_0) \int_\nu \alpha_\nu \, d\nu \tag{2.15}$$

where $\int \alpha_\nu \, d\nu$ is obtained from Eq. (2.10). Thus, from the definition, Eq. (2.15), $\int_\nu g(\nu, \nu_0) \, d\nu = 1$, where, as usual, the interval of integration is over the entire spectral line.

For pressures above 10–20 Torr, the line shape is dominated by *collision broadening* (or *pressure broadening*). It has been demonstrated that, for this case, the line shape is a Lorentz curve (see, for example, Lengyel, 1971).

$$g(\nu, \nu_0) = \frac{\Delta\nu}{2\pi} \frac{1}{[(\nu - \nu_0)^2 + (\Delta\nu/2)^2]} \tag{2.16}$$

Here, $\Delta\nu$ is the *line width* (see Fig. 2.7), given by

$$\Delta\nu = Z/\pi \tag{2.17}$$

where Z is the molecular collision frequency.

For absorption at line center, $\nu - \nu_0 = 0$, and, from Eqs. (2.15), (2.16), and (2.17),

$$\alpha_\nu = \frac{2}{\pi\,\Delta\nu} \int_\nu \alpha_\nu \, d\nu = \frac{2}{Z} \int_\nu \alpha_\nu \, d\nu$$

Substitute Eq. (2.10) into the above

$$\alpha_\nu = \frac{\lambda^2 A_{21}}{4\pi Z}\left(N_1 - \frac{g_1}{g_2} N_2\right) \tag{2.18}$$

Now, recalling our definition of *small-signal gain coefficient,* Eq. (2.4), and combining Eqs. (2.5) and (2.18), we have

$$G_0 = \frac{\lambda^2 A_{21}}{4\pi Z}\left(\frac{g_1}{g_2} N_2 - N_1\right) \tag{2.19}$$

In terms of the radiative lifetime, $\tau_{12} = 1/A_{21}$,

$$G_0 = \frac{\lambda^2}{4\pi\tau_{12} Z}\left(\frac{g_1}{g_2} N_2 - N_1\right) \tag{2.20}$$

Equation (2.20) is our desired result for *small-signal gain coefficient.*

For CO_2–N_2–H_2O or He lasers, the physical data necessary for evaluating Eq. (2.20) are as follows. From the experimental measurements of Gerry and Leonard (1966), $\lambda = 10.6\ \mu$m and $\tau_{12} = 5.38$ sec. The molecular collision frequency is

$$Z = \sum_i N_i \sigma_i \bar{V}_{CO_2-i} \tag{2.21}$$

where the summation is over all chemical species in the laser mixture, N_i is the number of molecules of species i, σ_i is the collision cross section for collisions between CO_2 and species i, and $\bar{V}_{CO_2-i}$ is the relative velocity between the two colliding particles.

$$\bar{V}_{CO_2-i} = \left[\frac{8\mathcal{R}T}{\pi}\left(\frac{M_{CO_2} + M_i}{M_{CO_2} M_i}\right)\right]^{1/2} \tag{2.22}$$

where M_{CO_2} and M_i are the molecular masses of CO_2 and i, respectively, and $\mathcal{R}$ is the universal gas constant. The collision cross sections in Eq. (2.21) are: $\sigma_{CO_2} = 1.30 \times 10^{-14}$ cm^2, $\sigma_{N_2} = 0.87 \times 10^{-14}$ cm^2, $\sigma_{He} = 0.37 \times 10^{-14}$ cm^2, and $\sigma_{H_2O} = 0.38 \times 10^{-14}$ cm^2.

Note that, for a given gas, the number densities N_i are proportional to pressure p whereas the collision frequency is proportional to $p/T^{1/2}$, where T is temperature. Hence, Eq. (2.20) indicates that, for oscillation at line center (which is the case for most lasers), G_0 is explicitly *independent* of pressure. However, the reader should note that, in the gasdynamic laser, the nonequilibrium properties of the nozzle expansion *are* dependent on p. Hence, Eq. (2.20) is *implicitly dependent* on p through the dependence of N_1 and N_2 on the nonequilibrium expansion.

Finally, note that, from Eq. (2.20), small-signal gain is *directly proportional to the population inversion,* and hence an experimental measurement of G_0 *is* a measurement of population inversion.

Chapter III

Thermodynamics and Vibrational Kinetics of the CO_2–N_2–H_2O *or* He *Gasdynamic Laser*

3.1 Molecular Properties of CO_2 and N_2

If your eyes were capable of operating on a microscopic scale, you would see that the air around you is composed of a fantastic number of molecules (about 2.7×10^{19} molecules per cubic centimeter), all moving with an average velocity slightly higher than the speed of sound in air, and where each molecule is colliding with its neighboring molecules at the rate of 10^{10} per second. At the same time, the molecule is rotating about some axis of rotation, and the atoms that make up the molecule are executing a vibratory motion along or across the internuclear axis. It is this vibration, along with the attendant vibrational energy, in which we are most interested here; in any existing laser in which CO_2 is the lasing molecule, the laser radiation is produced by transitions from one CO_2 vibrational energy level to another. Moreover, for CO_2–N_2 lasers, the vibrational energy of N_2 plays an essential role in creating the population inversion between these two CO_2 vibrational energy levels. Let us examine this process in detail.

CO_2 is a linear, triatomic molecule with the modes of vibration shown in Fig. 3.1. The first mode consists of a symmetric stretching along the internuclear axis; the fundamental frequency of this vibration is ν_1, and the mode is identified as mode ν_1. Mode ν_2 is a bending vibration in which the bending can occur in the plane of the paper (as shown) or perpendicular to the paper; in this sense mode ν_2 is really two modes of vibration with the same fundamental frequency ν_2, hence it is "doubly degenerate." Mode ν_3 is an asymmetric vibration along the internuclear axis, with fundamental frequency ν_3. N_2, also shown in Fig. 3.1, is a diatomic molecule; hence it has only one mode of vibration with fundamental frequency ν.

As stated in Chapter II, the vibrational energies of these molecules are quantized. Some of the specific allowed energy levels for both CO_2 and N_2 are shown in Fig. 3.2. Only the first few levels for each mode are shown, because these are the only levels of interest for a CO_2–N_2 laser. The two laser transitions that have been observed in CO_2 are also shown in this figure. The transition between the 001 and 100 levels yields laser radiation at 10.6 μm and is by far the strongest source of CO_2 laser radiation. The transition between the 001 and 020 levels is usually very weak for most contemporary laser designs and will not be considered here.

Note that each of these modes has its own ladder of quantized energy levels, with the triple-quantum number notation (v_1, v_2, v_3) for CO_2 to designate each level. CO_2 is the lasing molecule, and of particular importance is the (001) *upper laser level* in the ν_3 mode and the (100) *lower laser level* in the ν_1 mode. This laser transition takes place at a wavelength near 10.6 μm, with the precise wavelength depending on the particular rotational levels involved. In fact, note that each vibrational level has a series of closely spaced rotational levels superimposed on it, and the actual laser transition takes place between two distinct *vibration–rotation* levels.

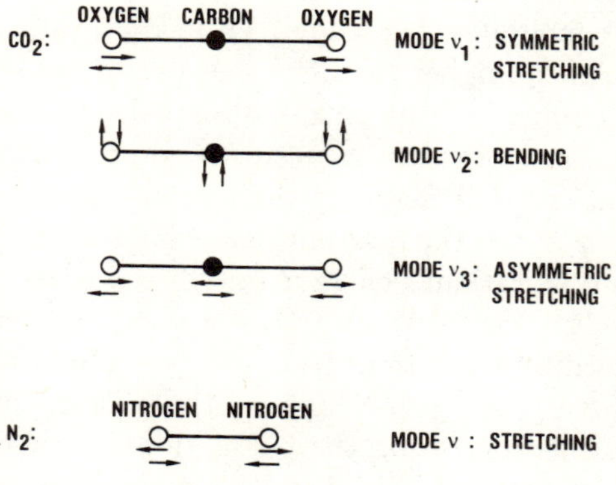

FIG. 3.1 Vibrational modes for carbon dioxide.

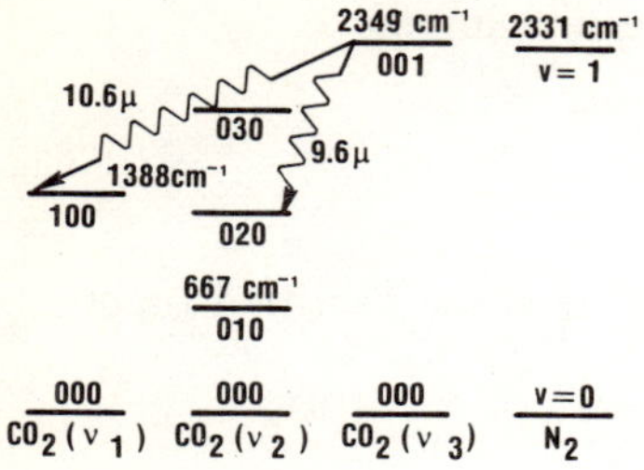

FIG. 3.2

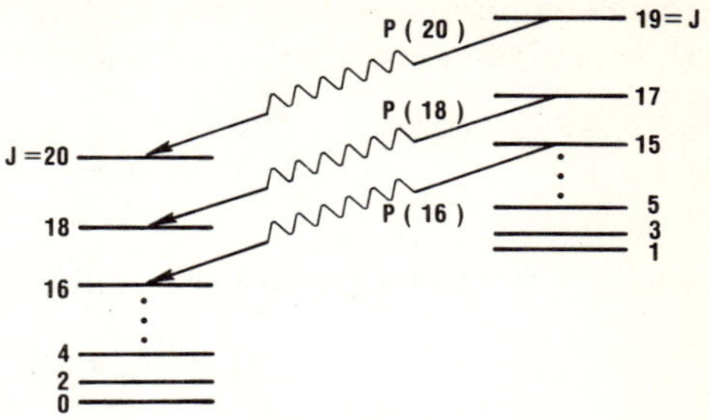

FIG. 3.3

FIG. 3.2 Low-lying vibrational energy levels in CO_2 and N_2, and the CO_2 laser transitions.

FIG. 3.3 P-Branch radiative transitions between vibration–rotation energy levels.

These levels are shown schematically in Fig. 3.3, where J denotes the rotational quantum number. A radiative transition that results in $\Delta J = -1$ is a member of the "P Branch," and several of the possible CO_2 laser transitions [P(20), P(18), P(16)] are shown in Fig. 3.3. If the gas translational temperature is near room temperature and the laser cavity is properly tuned, the P(20) transition is generally observed.

3.2 Vibrational Energy and Population Distribution

Now, let us turn down our microscopic vision and instead look at the overall vibrational energy of the gas from a macroscopic viewpoint. First, consider a unit mass of CO_2. The vibrational energy of this mass, $e_{\text{vib}_{CO_2}}$, is

$$e_{\text{vib}_{CO_2}} = \sum_i N_i \epsilon_i$$

where N_i is the number of CO_2 molecules per unit mass in the energy level ϵ_i; i.e., N_i is the population of the ϵ_i level, and the summation is over all the possible energy levels of CO_2. Similarly, for a unit mass of N_2,

$$e_{\text{vib}_{N_2}} = \sum_i N_i \epsilon_i$$

where N_i is now the population per unit mass of the N_2 energy level ϵ_i.

If the gas is left to itself over a period of time, with no perturbations or disturbances from the surroundings, the myriad molecular collisions within the system will drive the populations N_i, and hence $e_{\text{vib}_{CO_2}}$ and $e_{\text{vib}_{N_2}}$, to an equilibrium state. A major result of statistical thermodynamics gives the population distribution for a system in equilibrium as

$$N_i = N \frac{g_i \exp(-\epsilon_{i/kT})}{Q} \tag{3.1}$$

where N is the total number of particles, and Q is the partition function,

$$Q \equiv \sum_i g_i \exp(-\epsilon_{i/kT}).$$

This is called the *Boltzmann distribution* and is named after Ludwig Boltzmann, who was instrumental in the development of classical statistical mechanics in the late nineteenth century. In Eq. (3.1), k is the Boltzmann constant, equal to 1.38054×10^{-23} J/°K. Focusing directly on the vibrational energy and the vibrational population distribution, Eq. (3.1) gives, for a system of harmonic oscillators,

$$N_v = N \frac{e^{-vh\nu/kT}}{Q_{\text{vib}}} \tag{3.2}$$

where $Q_{\text{vib}} = (1 - e^{-h\nu/kT})^{-1}$, v is the vibrational quantum number, ν is the fundamental vibrational frequency, and h is Planck's constant, equal to 6.6256×10^{-34} Jsec. The combination $h\nu/k$ has dimensions of temperature and is called a characteristic vibrational temperature, $h\nu/k = \theta_\nu$. Hence, Eq. (3.2) becomes

$$N_v = Ne^{-v\theta_\nu/T}(1 - e^{-\theta_\nu/T}) \tag{3.3}$$

Again, remembering that $e_{\text{vib}} = \sum_i N_i\epsilon_i$, Eq. (3.3) leads directly to

$$e_{\text{vib}} = \left(\frac{\theta_\nu}{e^{\theta_\nu/T} - 1}\right)R \tag{3.4}$$

where R is the *specific* gas constant.

Equations (3.3) and (3.4) apply to a diatomic molecule with a single mode of vibrational energy, such as N_2. For N_2, $\theta_\nu = 3357$°K. For a polyatomic molecule, the previous equations can be extended, as discussed by Davidson (1962). The results, applied to CO_2, are as follows:

$$N_{v00} = N[\exp(-v\theta_{\nu_1}/T)]/Q_{\text{vib}_{CO_2}} \tag{3.5a}$$

$$N_{0v0} = N[\exp(-v\theta_{\nu_2}/T)]/Q_{\text{vib}_{CO_2}} \tag{3.5b}$$

$$N_{00v} = N[\exp(-v\theta_{\nu_3}/T)]/Q_{\text{vib}_{CO_2}} \tag{3.5c}$$

where

$$Q_{\text{vib}CO_2} = [1 - \exp(-\theta_{\nu_1}/T)]^{-1}[1 - \exp(-\theta_{\nu_2}/T)]^{-2} \times [1 - \exp(-\theta_{\nu_3}/T)]^{-1} \tag{3.6}$$

and $\theta_{\nu_1} = 1999°K$, $\theta_{\nu_2} = 960°K$, $\theta_{\nu_3} = 3383°K$. Equations (3.5a–c) give the population distribution within the ν_1, ν_2, and ν_3 modes of CO_2, respectively. The vibrational energy per unit mass of CO_2 is correspondingly

$$e_{\text{vib}CO_2} = \left(\frac{\theta_{\nu_1}}{\exp(\theta_{\nu_1}/T) - 1} + \frac{2\theta_{\nu_2}}{\exp(\theta_{\nu_2}/T) - 1} + \frac{\theta_{\nu_3}}{\exp(\theta_{\nu_3}/T) - 1}\right)R \tag{3.7}$$

Equations (3.1)–(3.7) hold for a gas in thermodynamic equilibrium—indeed, the basic structure of statistical thermodynamics (from which these equations are obtained) is hinged on a system in equilibrium. However, a laser gas is *not* in equilibrium. The population inversion that makes a laser work (see Fig. 2.2) is an inherent nonequilibrium situation. In a gasdynamic laser, all possible efforts are made to produce a highly *nonequilibrium* expansion through the supersonic nozzle. This is somewhat foreign to aerodynamicists, who are usually working hard to create equilibrium flows, such as in high temperature wind tunnels, so that the test gas is well defined, and in rocket nozzle expansions, so as to obtain the maximum specific impulse. In the case of the gasdynamic laser, however, the aerodynamicist must strive for a nozzle expansion with a large degree of vibrational nonequilibrium, as described in the following chapters. Why, then, have we bothered to obtain Eqs. (3.1)–(3.7)?

The answer is found in the fact that numerous types of vibrational nonequilibrium flows are closely approximated by a Boltzmann distribution over the vibrational energy levels but at a "temperature" different than the static (or translational) temperature of the gas. That is, for many nonequilibrium situations, Eq. (3.2) gives a reasonable prediction of the population distribution but with the temperature replaced by a *vibrational* temperature T_{vib}.

$$N_v = N \exp(-v\theta_\nu/T_{\text{vib}})/Q_{\text{vib}} \tag{3.8}$$

where

$$Q_{\text{vib}} = [1 - \exp(-\theta_\nu/T_{\text{vib}})]^{-1}.$$

Consistent with this assumption of a local Boltzmann distribution is the nonequilibrium vibrational energy obtained from an equation similar to Eq. (3.4):

$$\text{nonequilibrium } e_{\text{vib}} = \theta_\nu R/[\exp(\theta_\nu/T_{\text{vib}}) - 1] \tag{3.9}$$

Indeed, as we shall soon see, e_{vib} is the fundamental quantity usually obtained in a nonequilibrium flow analysis, and T_{vib} is subsequently defined by Eq. (3.9). The concept of a vibrational temperature is extremely useful in gasdynamic laser analyses, as described in subsequent sections.

3.3 Vibrational Kinetics

Let us once again think of the laser gas as a collection of molecules in motion. These molecules are colliding with each other on a regular basis. During any of these collisions, there is a finite probability that some of the translational energy of one molecule will be transferred as vibrational energy to the other—this is called a *T–V transfer*. Also, if one of the colliding molecules already has some vibrational energy, then there is a finite probability that this vibrational energy will be transferred as vibrational energy to the other molecule—this is called a *V–V transfer*. Now, referring again to the energy level diagram in Fig. 3.2, a number of different molecular energy transfer processes can be anticipated between the various modes of CO_2 and between CO_2 and N_2. These processes are nicely catalogued by Taylor and Bitterman (1969) and fall within three general types: T–V processes, V–V processes (intermolecular), and V–V processes (intramolecular). The detailed energy transfer processes can be written as kinetic reactions (analogous to chemical reaction equations) as follows:

T–V Processes

$$CO_2^*\ (\nu_2) + M \rightleftarrows CO_2 + M + 667\ \text{cm}^{-1} \tag{3.10}$$

$$N_2^* + M \rightleftarrows N_2 + M + 2331\ \text{cm}^{-1} \tag{3.11}$$

V–V Process (intermolecular)

$$CO_2^*\ (\nu_3) + N_2 \rightleftarrows CO_2 + N_2^* + 18\ \text{cm}^{-1} \tag{3.12}$$

V–V Processes (intramolecular)

$$CO_2^*\ (\nu_3) + M \rightleftarrows CO_2^{***}\ (\nu_2) + M + 416\ \text{cm}^{-1} \tag{3.13}$$

$$CO_2^*\ (\nu_1) + M \rightleftarrows CO_2^{**}\ (\nu_2) + M + 102\ \text{cm}^{-1} \tag{3.14}$$

In the above equations, M stands for a collision partner that can be CO_2, N_2, H_2O, or He. The asterisks indicate the vibrational level in a given mode. For example, Eq. (3.13) reads that CO_2 in the (001) level of the ν_3 mode, after colliding with a molecule of species M, will yield CO_2 in the (030) level of the ν_2 mode, and the complete interaction process will give up 416 cm^{-1} of energy to the translational and rotational motion of the molecules. Also, examining Eqs. (3.10)–(3.14) along with Fig. 3.2, the following are noted:

(a) The 001 level of CO_2 and the $v = 1$ level of N_2 are almost the same energy, separated by only 18 cm^{-1}; they are near-resonant. This implies that the process given by Eq. (3.12) is extremely rapid. This reaction is called the "pumping" reaction.

(b) The population of the upper laser level (001) is dependent on the population of N_2 in $v = 1$ through the pumping reaction, Eq. (3.12). In addition, it also depends on the rate of reaction (3.13) and on the rate of laser power extraction, which tends to deplete the 001 level.

(c) The 100 and 020 levels of CO_2 are relatively close; moreover, because of the known Fermi resonance between these two levels, reaction (3.14) is very fast.

(d) The population of the lower laser level (100) is basically dependent on the rate of laser power extraction, which tends to fill the level, and on the population of the 020 level via reaction (3.14).

For the analysis of gasdynamic laser performance, the points (a)–(d) lead to simplified models of the vibrational kinetic processes. These models will be developed in subsequent sections.

3.4 Vibrational Rate Equations

An important objective of almost any gasdynamic laser analysis is to obtain the populations of the upper and lower laser levels; for CO_2–N_2–H_2O or He mixtures, this means N_{001} and N_{100}, respectively. These values define the population inversion necessary to calculate the small-signal gain coefficient, Eq. (2.20), and are required for a detailed calculation of laser power extraction. In turn, N_{001} and N_{100} are at least dependent on the rate of reactions (3.10)–(3.14), i.e., on *how fast* molecules are entering or leaving various energy levels. Therefore, at first glance, equations describing the time rate of change of populations such as dN_{001}/dt and dN_{100}/dt appear necessary. However, if such *rate equations* were obtained for the population of *all* energy levels shown in Fig. 3.2, our analysis would be encumbered with unnecessary detail and complexity. Indeed, such an analysis would be impossible at the present time due to the lack of rate data for some of the detailed transitions that would have to be included. For example, what is the rate of the V–V transition between the 020 and 010 levels? It is known to be extremely fast, but what is the actual value for this rate? Such information is lacking, but, fortunately, we do not need it. The reasons are given below.

First, the very fact that intramode V–V transfers, such as 020–010, are extremely fast (due to near-resonance of the vibrational levels within any single mode) insures that a near Boltzmann distribution exists locally within that mode. Hence it is reasonable to assume that each mode is in equilibrium within itself but not with each other. It follows that vibrational temperatures for each CO_2 mode and for N_2 can be defined from the vibrational energy for each mode. Let E_1, E_2, E_3, and E_4 be the energy for the ν_1, ν_2, and ν_3 modes of CO_2, and for N_2, respectively. Let T_1, T_2, T_3, and T_4 be the corresponding vibrational temperatures, all different from each other and from the static temperature T of the gas. This nomenclature is similar to that used by Munjee (1972).

Secondly, the Fermi resonance between the (100) and (020) is believed to be very strong; hence reaction (3.14) is extremely fast. Thus, the ν_1 and ν_2 modes are closely coupled and are assumed to be in local equilibrium with each other. As a result, we can deal with the combined vibrational energies of these modes, E_{12}, where $E_{12} = E_1 + 2E_2$ (recall that the ν_2 mode is doubly degenerate). Also, $T_{12} = T_1 = T_2$. However, it should be noted that recent information has raised some questions about the local equilibrium normally assumed between the ν_1 and ν_2 modes. Specifically, Rosser *et al.* (1972) present data that indicate that such equilibrium may not exist for all laser conditions. This contention is further supported by Bulthius (1973), who presents a measured rate for energy transfer from the (100) to (020) levels that is an order of magnitude slower than previously reported values and prompts a comment that the vibrational temperatures of the ν_1 and ν_2 modes are not always the same, particularly during peak power extraction. On the other hand, De Temple *et al.* (1973) countered these contentions by presenting measurements for the decay rate of CO_2 (100) that are an order of magnitude faster than those of Rosser *et al.* (1972). De Temple *et al.* (1973) feel that their measurements are more representative of the intrinsic V–V relaxation process, whereas those of Rosser *et al.* (1972) are more characteristic of a V–T process under the influence of a perturbing radiation field. On the other hand, very recent measurements by Murray (1974) seem to support the slower rate and indicate that equilibrium does not always exist between the ν_1 and ν_2 modes. This matter, albeit an important one, is still in a state of flux; until it is resolved, the assumption of local equilibrium between the ν_1 and ν_2 modes appears to be the only logical recourse for gasdynamic laser calculations.

As a result, the detailed energy level diagram of Fig. 3.2 can be modeled as shown in Fig. 3.4, where the ν_1 and ν_2 modes are combined. Transfers into and out of the combined mode occur via reactions (3.10) and (3.13). This model is the same as that described by Munjee (1972). In this model, the fundamental quantities are not the populations N_i, but rather the energies E_{12}, E_3, and E_4 of the combined $(\nu_1 + 2\nu_2)$ mode, the ν_3 mode, and N_2, respectively. The time rates of net energy transfer into or out of these modes are given by dE_{12}/dt, dE_3/dt, and dE_4/dt. The expressions giving these time derivatives are the *rate equations for vibrational energy transfer*. Let us proceed to derive and list these rate equations.

First, consider two colliding molecules. The probability that the collision will result in a transfer of vibrational energy from one molecule to another depends on such details as the relative velocity between the centers of mass of the molecules, the distance of closest approach, and the actual force field and molecular structure of each molecule. Most collisions do not yield a vibrational energy transfer; usually, one collision out of a thousand (or more) yields such a transfer. Hence, the *probability* that any *single* collision will result in a T–V or V–V transfer is usually much less than unity, say 10^{-3} or 10^{-4}.

Let us be more specific for the CO_2–N_2 system shown in Fig. 3.4. Consider just the N_2 vibrational energy per unit mass E_4 and consider a N_2 molecule colliding with a CO_2, N_2, H_2O, or He molecule (designated as species i). The following *transition probabilities* are defined:

$\overset{10}{P}(\mathrm{N}, i)$ = probability of T–V transition from $v = 1$ to $v = 0$ level of N_2 due to a collision with a molecule of species i.

$\overset{j,j-1}{P}(\mathrm{N}, i)$ = probability of T–V transition from the j to the $j - 1$ level of N_2 due to a collision with a molecule of species i.

$\underset{01}{\overset{10}{Q}}(\mathrm{N, C3})\,(m_0/N_{CO_2})$ = probability of V–V transition from the $v = 1$ to the $v = 0$ level of N_2 due to a collision with a CO_2 molecule that simultaneously experiences a transition from the $\nu_3 = 0$ to the $\nu_3 = 1$ level.

$\underset{k,k+1}{\overset{j,j-1}{Q}}(\mathrm{N, C3})\,(m_k/N_{CO_2})$ = probability of V–V transition from the j to the $j - 1$ level of N_2 due to a collision with a CO_2 molecule that simultaneously experiences a transition from the k to the $k + 1$ level.

In the above, m_0 and m_k represent the population of the 0th and kth level

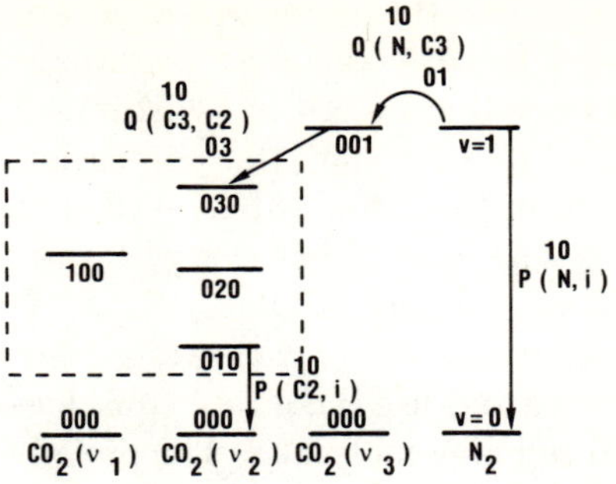

FIG. 3.4 A vibrational kinetic model for CO_2–N_2. (After Munjee, 1972.)

of CO_2 (ν_3), respectively, and N_{CO_2} is the total number of CO_2 molecules. The weighting factor (m_k/N_{CO_2}) is considered to be an integral part of the V–V transition probability, because the opportunity for a single N_2 molecule to exchange vibrational energy with a CO_2 molecule in the kth level *depends* on the number of CO_2 molecules that are *available* in the kth level. The transition probabilities for the reverse processes,

$$\overset{01}{P}(N, i), \quad \overset{j-1,j}{P}(\mathrm{N}, i), \quad \overset{01}{\underset{10}{Q}}(\mathrm{N}, \mathrm{C3})\,(m_1/N_{CO_2}), \quad \overset{j-1,j}{\underset{k+1,k}{Q}}(\mathrm{N}, \mathrm{C3})\,(m_{k+1}/N_{CO_2}),$$

are similarly defined.

Let $n_0, n_1, \ldots, n_i, \ldots$ be the populations of the $v = 0, 1, \ldots, i, \ldots$ levels of N_2. Also, let $Z_{\mathrm{N}i}$ be the collision frequency (collisions per second) of one N_2 molecule with the i molecules (i = N_2, CO_2, H_2O, He). Now consider the $v = 1$ level of N_2. The number of T–V transitions per second *into* this level from $v = 0$ due to collisions with other N_2 molecules is

$$\left\{\begin{array}{l}\text{Number of collisions}\\ \text{per second of } N_2\\ \text{molecules in the}\\ v = 0 \text{ level with}\\ \text{other } N_2 \text{ molecules}\end{array}\right\} \times \left\{\begin{array}{l}\text{Transition probability}\\ \text{from } v = 0 \text{ to } v = 1,\\ \text{i.e., number of}\\ \text{transitions ``per}\\ \text{collision''}\end{array}\right\}$$

$$= (n_0 Z_{\mathrm{NN}})[\overset{01}{P}(\mathrm{N}, \mathrm{N})]$$

Similarly, the number of T–V transitions per second *out* of this level from $v = 1$ to $v = 0$ due to collisions with other N_2 molecules is $(n_1 Z_{\mathrm{NN}})[\overset{10}{P}(\mathrm{N}, \mathrm{N})]$. A relation between $\overset{10}{P}(\mathrm{N}, \mathrm{N})$ and $\overset{01}{P}(\mathrm{N}, \mathrm{N})$ can now be obtained from the *principle of detailed balancing.* If the system is in equilibrium, the forward and reverse processes take place an equal number of times over any given interval of time. Hence,

$$n_0 Z_{\mathrm{NN}} \overset{01}{P}(\mathrm{N, N}) = n_1 Z_{\mathrm{NN}} \overset{10}{P}(\mathrm{N, N}).$$

Therefore,

$$\overset{01}{P}(\mathrm{N, N}) = (n_1/n_0) \overset{10}{P}(\mathrm{N, N})$$

However, for a system in equilibrium, n_1/n_0 is given by the Boltzmann distribution, Eq. (3.2):

$$n_1/n_0 = \exp(-h\nu/kT) = \exp(-\theta_4/T)$$

where T is the temperature of the system, and $\theta_4 = h\nu/k$ is the characteristic vibrational temperature for N_2. Thus,

$$\overset{01}{P}(\mathrm{N, N}) = \exp(-\theta_4/T) \overset{10}{P}(\mathrm{N, N}) \tag{3.15}$$

Similarly

$$\overset{j-1,j}{P}(\mathrm{N, N}) = \exp(-\theta_4/T) \overset{j,j-1}{P}(\mathrm{N, N}) \tag{3.16}$$

In addition, for a simple harmonic oscillator,

$$\overset{j,j-1}{P}(\mathrm{N, N}) = j \overset{10}{P}(\mathrm{N, N}) \tag{3.17}$$

Combining Eqs. (3.16) and (3.17),

$$\overset{j-1,j}{P}(\mathrm{N, N}) = j \exp(-\theta_4/T) \overset{10}{P}(\mathrm{N, N}) \tag{3.18}$$

For V–V transitions, the principle of detailed balancing gives

$$n_0 Z_{\mathrm{NC}} \underset{10}{\overset{01}{Q}}(\mathrm{N, C3}) m_1/N_{\mathrm{CO_2}} = n_1 Z_{\mathrm{NC}} \underset{01}{\overset{10}{Q}}(\mathrm{N, C3}) m_0/N_{\mathrm{CO_2}}$$

$$\underset{10}{\overset{01}{Q}}(\mathrm{N, C3}) = (n_1/n_0) \underset{01}{\overset{10}{Q}}(\mathrm{N, C3}) m_0/m_1 \tag{3.19}$$

However, $n_1/n_0 = \exp(-\theta_4/T)$ and $m_0/m_1 = \exp(\theta_3/T)$. Thus, Eq. (3.19) becomes

$$\underset{10}{\overset{01}{Q}}(\mathrm{N, C3}) = \exp[(\theta_3 - \theta_4)/T] \underset{01}{\overset{10}{Q}}(\mathrm{N, C3}) \tag{3.20}$$

Similarly,

$$\underset{k+1,k}{\overset{j-1,j}{Q}}(\mathrm{N, C3}) = \exp[(\theta_3 - \theta_4)/T] \underset{k,k+1}{\overset{j,j-1}{Q}}(\mathrm{N, C3}) \tag{3.21}$$

Also, as stated by Schwartz *et al.* (1952),

$$\overset{j,j+1}{\underset{k+1,k}{Q}}(\mathrm{N, C3}) = (j+1)(k+1)\overset{01}{\underset{10}{Q}}(\mathrm{N, C3}) \tag{3.22}$$

and

$$\overset{j,j-1}{\underset{k,k+1}{Q}}(\mathrm{N, C3}) = j(k+1)\overset{10}{\underset{01}{Q}}(\mathrm{N, C3})$$

which, from Eq. (3.20), becomes

$$\overset{j,j-1}{\underset{k,k+1}{Q}}(\mathrm{N, C3}) = j(k+1)\exp[(\theta_4 - \theta_3)/T]\overset{01}{\underset{10}{Q}}(\mathrm{N, C3}) \tag{3.23}$$

Keeping Eqs. (3.15)–(3.23) in mind, now consider the total vibrational energy of N_2, E_4. For simplicity later on, consider a unit mass of N_2; hence *E_4 is the N_2 vibrational energy per unit mass.* Vibrational energy transfers, both T–V and V–V, that increase the vibrational quantum number V, $\Delta V = +1$, serve to increase E_4; conversely, transfers that result in $\Delta V = -1$ decrease E_4. The net time rate of change of E_4 is

$$\begin{aligned} dE_4/dt = h\nu[&\text{T–V transfers per second yielding } \Delta V = +1) \\ &- (\text{T–V transfers per second yielding } \Delta V = -1) \\ &+ (\text{V–V transfers per second yielding } \Delta V = +1) \\ &- (\text{V–V transfers per second yielding } \Delta V = -1)] \end{aligned} \tag{3.24}$$

Consider each term in Eq. (3.24) separately.

$$\left\{\begin{matrix}\text{T–V transfers per second} \\ \text{yielding } \Delta V = +1 \text{ due} \\ \text{to collisions with } N_2\end{matrix}\right\}$$

$$\begin{aligned} &= n_0 Z_{NN} \overset{01}{P}(\mathrm{N, N}) + n_1 Z_{NN} \overset{12}{P}(\mathrm{N, N}) \\ &\quad + n_2 Z_{NN} \overset{23}{P}(\mathrm{N, N}) + \cdots + n_j Z_{NN} \overset{j,j+1}{P}(\mathrm{N, N}) + \cdots \\ &= Z_{NN} \sum_{j=0}^{\infty} n_j \overset{j,j+1}{P}(\mathrm{N, N}) \\ &= Z_{NN} \sum_{j=0}^{\infty} n_j \exp(-\theta_4/T) \overset{j+1,j}{P}(\mathrm{N, N}) \\ &= Z_{NN} \sum_{j=0}^{\infty} n_j \exp(-\theta_4/T)(j+1) \overset{10}{P}(\mathrm{N, N}) \\ &= Z_{NN} \exp(-\theta_4/T) \overset{10}{P}(\mathrm{N, N}) \left[\sum_{j=0}^{\infty} j n_j + \sum_{j=0}^{\infty} n_j\right] \end{aligned} \tag{3.25}$$

However,

$$\sum_{j=0}^{\infty} jn_j = n_1 + 2n_2 + 3n_3 + \cdots$$

$$= n_0\left(\frac{n_1}{n_0} + 2\frac{n_2}{n_1}\frac{n_1}{n_0} + 3\frac{n_3}{n_2}\frac{n_2}{n_1}\frac{n_1}{n_0} + \cdots\right) \tag{3.26}$$

From the Boltzmann distribution,

$$\frac{n_1}{n_0} = \exp(-\theta_4/T)\,;\ \frac{n_2}{n_1}\frac{n_1}{n_0} = [\exp(-\theta_4/T)]^2 = \exp(-2\theta_4/T)\,; \quad \text{etc.}$$

Hence, Eq. (3.26) becomes

$$\sum_{j=0}^{\infty} jn_j = n_0[\exp(-\theta_4/T) + 2\exp(-2\theta_4/T) + 3\exp(-3\theta_4/T) + \cdots]$$

$$= n_0 \exp(-\theta_4/T)[1 + 2\exp(-\theta_4/T) + 3\exp(-2\theta_4/T) + \cdots] \tag{3.27}$$

Using the series expansion

$$[1 - \exp(-\theta_4/T)]^{-2} = 1 + 2\exp(-\theta_4/T) + 3\exp(-2\theta_4/T) + \cdots$$

Eq. (3.27) becomes

$$\sum_{j=0}^{\infty} jn_j = n_0 \exp(-\theta_4/T)[1 - \exp(-\theta_4/T)]^{-2} \tag{3.28}$$

Now, from the Boltzmann distribution, Eq. (3.3),

$$n_0 = N_{N_2}[1 - \exp(-\theta_4/T)] \tag{3.29}$$

Substituting Eq. (3.29) into Eq. (3.28),

$$\sum_{j=0}^{\infty} jn_j = N_{N_2}[1 - \exp(-\theta_4/T)]\exp(-\theta_4/T)[1 - \exp(-\theta_4/T)]^{-2}$$

$$= N_{N_2} \exp(-\theta_4/T)[1 - \exp(-\theta_4/T)]^{-1}$$

$$= N_{N_2}/[\exp(\theta_4/T) - 1) \tag{3.30}$$

From Eq. (3.4), the total vibrational energy per unit mass of N_2 is

$$E_4 \equiv E_{N_2} = [\theta_4/(\exp(\theta_4/T) - 1)]R_{N_2} \tag{3.31}$$

where R_{N_2} is the specific gas constant for N_2. Again note that E_4 is in general a nonequilibrium value, hence T is the vibrational temperature T_4. From Eq. (3.31),

$$\exp(\theta_4/T) - 1 = \theta_4 R_{N_2}/E_4 \tag{3.32}$$

Substituting Eq. (3.32) into Eq. (3.30),

$$\sum_{j=0}^{\infty} jn_j = N_{N_2}E_4/\theta_4 R_{N_2} \tag{3.33}$$

Also

$$\sum_{j=0}^{\infty} n_j = N_{N_2} \tag{3.34}$$

Substituting Eqs. (3.33) and (3.34) into Eq. (3.25),

$$\left\{\begin{matrix}\text{T–V transfers per second}\\ \text{yielding } \Delta V = +1 \text{ due to}\\ \text{collisions with } N_2\end{matrix}\right\} = Z_{NN}\overset{10}{P}(N, N)\exp(-\theta_4/T)N_{N_2}\left(\frac{E_4}{\theta_4 R_{N_2}} + 1\right)$$

In a similar fashion

$$\left\{\begin{matrix}\text{T–V transfers per second}\\ \text{yielding } \Delta V = +1 \text{ due to}\\ \text{collisions with } CO_2\end{matrix}\right\} = Z_{NC}\overset{10}{P}(N, C)\exp(-\theta_4/T)N_{N_2}\left(\frac{E_4}{\theta_4 R_{N_2}} + 1\right)$$

$$\left\{\begin{matrix}\text{T–V transfers per second}\\ \text{yielding } \Delta V = +1 \text{ due to}\\ \text{collisions with } H_2O \text{ or He}\end{matrix}\right\} = Z_{NH}\overset{10}{P}(N, H)\exp(-\theta_4/T)N_{N_2}\left(\frac{E_4}{\theta_4 R_{N_2}} + 1\right)$$

Thus, the first term of Eq. (3.24) is

$$\left\{\begin{matrix}\text{T–V transfers per second}\\ \text{yielding } \Delta V = +1\end{matrix}\right\} = [Z_{NN}\overset{10}{P}(N, N) + Z_{NC}\overset{10}{P}(N, C) + Z_{NH}\overset{10}{P}(N, H)] \times N_{N_2}\exp(-\theta_4/T)\left(\frac{E_4}{\theta_4 R_{N_2}} + 1\right) \tag{3.35}$$

Moving to the second term of Eq. (3.24), we have

$$\begin{aligned}\left\{\begin{matrix}\text{T–V transfers per second}\\ \text{yielding } \Delta V = -1 \text{ due}\\ \text{to collisions with } N_2\end{matrix}\right\} &= n_1 Z_{NN}\overset{10}{P}(N, N) + n_2 Z_{NN}\overset{21}{P}(N, N) + \cdots + n_j Z_{NN}\overset{j,j-1}{P}(N, N) + \cdots \\ &= \sum_{j=1}^{\infty} n_j Z_{NN}\overset{j,j-1}{P}(N, N) \\ &= Z_{NN}\sum_{j=1}^{\infty} jn_j\overset{10}{P}(N, N) \\ &= Z_{NN}\overset{10}{P}(N, N)\sum_{j=1}^{\infty} jn_j\end{aligned}$$

However, from Eq. (3.33),

$$\sum_{j=1}^{\infty} jn_j = \sum_{j=0}^{\infty} jn_j = N_{N_2}E_4/\theta_4 R_{N_2}$$

$$\begin{Bmatrix}\text{T–V transfers per second} \\ \text{yielding } \Delta V = -1 \text{ due} \\ \text{to collisions with } N_2\end{Bmatrix} = Z_{NN}\overset{10}{P}(N, N) N_{N_2}E_4/\theta_4 R_{N_2}$$

Similar expressions are obtained for collisions with CO_2 and H_2O or He. Thus, the second term in Eq. (3.24) is

$$\begin{Bmatrix}\text{T–V transfers per second} \\ \text{yielding } \Delta V = -1\end{Bmatrix} = [Z_{NN}\overset{10}{P}(N, N) + Z_{NC}\overset{10}{P}(N, C) + Z_{NH}\overset{10}{P}(N, H)]N_{N_2}\frac{E_4}{\theta_4 R_{N_2}} \tag{3.36}$$

Considering the third term in Eq. (3.24)

{V–V transfers per second yielding $\Delta V = +1$ due to collisions with CO_2}

$$= \left[n_0 Z_{NC} \overset{01}{\underset{10}{Q}}(N, C3)\frac{m_1}{N_{CO_2}} + n_0 Z_{NC}\overset{01}{\underset{21}{Q}}(N, C3)\frac{m_2}{N_{CO_2}} + \cdots\right]$$

$$+ \left[n_1 Z_{NC}\overset{12}{\underset{10}{Q}}(N, C3)\frac{m_1}{N_{CO_2}} + n_1 Z_{NC}\overset{12}{\underset{21}{Q}}(N, C3)\frac{m_2}{N_{CO_2}} + \cdots\right] + \cdots$$

$$= n_0 Z_{NC}\sum_{j=0}^{\infty}\overset{01}{\underset{j+1,j}{Q}}(N, C3)\frac{m_{j+1}}{N_{CO_2}} + n_1 Z_{NC}\sum_{j=0}^{\infty}\overset{12}{\underset{j+1,j}{Q}}(N, C3)\frac{m_{j+1}}{N_{CO_2}} + \cdots$$

$$= \sum_{k=0}^{\infty} n_k Z_{NC}\sum_{j=0}^{\infty}\overset{k,k+1}{\underset{j+1,j}{Q}}(N, C3)\frac{m_{j+1}}{N_{CO_2}}$$

$$= \sum_{k=0}^{\infty} n_k Z_{NC}(k+1)\sum_{j=0}^{\infty}(j+1)\overset{01}{\underset{10}{Q}}(N, C3)\frac{m_{j+1}}{N_{CO_2}}$$

$$= \frac{Z_{NC}}{N_{CO_2}}\overset{01}{\underset{10}{Q}}(N, C3)\sum_{k=0}^{\infty}(k+1)n_k\sum_{j=0}^{\infty}(j+1)m_{j+1} \tag{3.37}$$

However, from a derivation exactly the same as that leading to Eq. (3.33),

$$\sum_{j=0}^{\infty}(j+1)m_{j+1} = \sum_{j=0}^{\infty} jm_j = N_{CO_2}E_3/\theta_3 R_{CO_2} \tag{3.38}$$

where E_3 is the vibrational energy within the ν_3 mode of CO_2 per unit mass of CO_2, R_{CO_2} is the specific gas constant for CO_2, and θ_3 is the characteristic vibrational temperature for mode ν_3. Also, note that

$$\sum_{k=0}^{\infty} (k+1)n_k = \sum_{k=0}^{\infty} kn_k + \sum_{k=0}^{\infty} n_k = \frac{N_{N_2}E_4}{\theta_4 R_{N_2}} + N_{N_2} = N_{N_2}\left(\frac{E_4}{\theta_4 R_{N_2}} + 1\right) \tag{3.39}$$

Substituting Eqs. (3.38) and (3.39) into Eq. (3.37), we obtain the third term of Eq. (3.24)

$$\left\{\begin{array}{l}\text{V–V transfers per second}\\ \text{yielding } \Delta V = +1 \text{ due}\\ \text{to collisions with } CO_2\end{array}\right\} = Z_{NC}Q\overset{01}{\underset{10}{(N, C3)}}N_{N_2}\left(\frac{E_4}{\theta_4 R_{N_2}} + 1\right)\frac{E_3}{\theta_3 R_{CO_2}} \tag{3.40}$$

Considering the last term in Eq. (3.24), we have

{V–V transfers per second yielding $\Delta V = -1$ due to collisions with CO_2}

$$= n_1 Z_{NC}Q\overset{10}{\underset{01}{(N, C3)}}\frac{m_0}{N_{CO_2}}$$

$$+ n_1 Z_{NC}Q\overset{10}{\underset{12}{(N, C3)}}\frac{m_1}{N_{CO_2}} + \cdots + n_2 Z_{NC}Q\overset{21}{\underset{01}{(N, C3)}}\frac{m_0}{N_{CO_2}}$$

$$+ n_2 Z_{NC}Q\overset{21}{\underset{12}{(N, C3)}}\frac{m_1}{N_{CO_2}} + \cdots$$

$$= \sum_{k=1}^{\infty} n_k Z_{NC} \sum_{j=0}^{\infty} Q\overset{k,k-1}{\underset{j,j+1}{(N, C3)}}\frac{m_j}{N_{CO_2}}$$

$$= \sum_{k=1}^{\infty} n_k Z_{NC} \sum_{j=0}^{\infty} k(j+1)\exp[(\theta_4 - \theta_3)/T]Q\overset{01}{\underset{10}{(N, C3)}}\frac{m_j}{N_{CO_2}}$$

$$= \frac{Z_{NC}}{N_{CO_2}}\exp[(\theta_4 - \theta_3)/T]Q\overset{01}{\underset{10}{(N, C3)}}\sum_{k=1}^{\infty} kn_k \sum_{j=0}^{\infty}(j+1)m_j \tag{3.41}$$

However, as before,

$$\sum_{j=0}^{\infty}(j+1)m_j = \sum_{j=0}^{\infty} jm_j + \sum_{j=0}^{\infty} m_j = N_{CO_2}\left(\frac{E_3}{\theta_3 R_{CO_2}} + 1\right)$$

Also,

$$\sum_{k=1}^{\infty} kn_k = N_{N_2}E_4/\theta_4 R_{N_2}$$

Substituting the above into Eq. (3.41), we obtain the last term of Eq. (3.24)

{V–V transfers per second yielding $\Delta V = -1$ due to collisions with CO_2}

$$= Z_{NC} \exp[(\theta_4 - \theta_3)/T] Q(\overset{01}{N}, \underset{10}{C3}) \frac{N_{N_2} E_4}{\theta_4 R_{N_2}} \left(\frac{E_3}{\theta_3 R_{CO_2}} + 1 \right) \tag{3.42}$$

For the complete rate equation, substituting Eqs. (3.35), (3.36), (3.40), and (3.42) into Eq. (3.24), we have

$$\begin{aligned}\frac{dE_4}{dt} = h\nu N_{N_2} \Big\{ & [Z_{NN} P(\overset{10}{N}, N) + Z_{NC} P(\overset{10}{N}, C) + Z_{NH} P(\overset{10}{N}, H)] \\ & \times \left[\exp(-\theta_4/T) \left(\frac{E_4}{\theta_4 R_{N_2}} + 1 \right) - \frac{E_4}{\theta_4 R_{N_2}} \right] + Z_{NC} Q(\overset{01}{N}, \underset{10}{C3}) \\ & \times \left[\left(\frac{E_4}{\theta_4 R_{N_2}} + 1 \right) \frac{E_3}{\theta_3 R_{CO_2}} - \exp[(\theta_4 - \theta_3)/T] \left(\frac{E_4}{\theta_4 R_{N_2}} \right) \right. \\ & \left. \times \left(\frac{E_3}{\theta_3 R_{CO_2}} + 1 \right) \right] \Big\} \end{aligned} \tag{3.43}$$

However,

$$h\nu N_{N_2} = (h\nu/k)(N_{N_2} k) = \theta_4 R_{N_2}$$

because N_{N_2} is the number of N_2 molecules per unit mass, k is the gas constant per molecule; hence $N_{N_2}k$ is the gas constant per unit mass, i.e., R_{N_2}. Thus, Eq. (3.43) becomes

$$\begin{aligned}\frac{dE_4}{dt} = & [Z_{NN} P(\overset{10}{N}, N) + Z_{NC} P(\overset{10}{N}, C) + Z_{NH} P(\overset{10}{N}, H] \\ & \times [\exp(-\theta_4/T)(E_4 + \theta_4 R_{N_2}) - E_4] + Z_{NC} Q(\overset{01}{N}, \underset{10}{C3}) \\ & \times \left[(E_4 + \theta_4 R_{N_2}) \frac{E_3}{\theta_3 R_{CO_2}} - \exp[(\theta_4 - \theta_3)/T] E_4 \left(\frac{E_3}{\theta_3 R_{CO_2}} + 1 \right) \right] \end{aligned} \tag{3.44}$$

Referring to Fig. 3.4, recall that E_4 is the local nonequilibrium, vibrational energy per unit mass of N_2, and Eq. (3.44) gives the time rate of change of this nonequilibrium energy. Also, recall that Eq. (3.44) is based on the assumption of a local Boltzmann distribution within N_2. The analogous rate equations for the vibrational energy of the combined ν_1 and ν_2 modes per unit mass of CO_2, E_{12}, and for the energy for the ν_3 mode, E_3, are given by Munjee (1972). These equations can be derived in a similar fashion as the above analysis for dE_4/dt, with the results

$$
\begin{aligned}
\frac{dE_{12}}{dt} &= 2\left[Z_{CC}P\left(\overset{10}{C2}, C\right) + Z_{CH}P\left(\overset{10}{C2}, H\right) + Z_{CN}P\left(\overset{10}{C2}, N\right)\right] \\
&\quad \times \left[\exp(-\theta_2/T)\theta_2 R_{CO_2} - E_2(1 - \exp(-\theta_2/T))\right] \\
&\quad + 3\theta_2 R_{CO_2}\left[Z_{CC}Q_C\left(\overset{03}{C2}, \underset{10}{C3}\right) + Z_{CH}Q_H\left(\overset{03}{C2}, \underset{10}{C3}\right)\right. \\
&\quad \left. + Z_{CN}Q_N\left(\overset{03}{C2}, \underset{10}{C3}\right)\right]\left[\left(\frac{E_2}{\theta_2 R_{CO_2}} + 1\right)^3\left(\frac{E_3}{\theta_3 R_{CO_2}}\right)\right. \\
&\quad \left. - \exp[(3\theta_2 - \theta_3)/T]\left(\frac{E_3}{\theta_3 R_{CO_2}} + 1\right)\left(\frac{E_2}{\theta_2 R_{CO_2}}\right)^3\right]
\end{aligned} \tag{3.45}
$$

$$
\begin{aligned}
\frac{dE_3}{dt} &= \left[Z_{CC}Q_C\left(\overset{03}{C2}, \underset{10}{C3}\right) + Z_{CH}Q_H\left(\overset{03}{C2}, \underset{10}{C3}\right) + Z_{CN}Q_N\left(\overset{03}{C2}, \underset{10}{C3}\right)\right] \\
&\quad \times \left[\exp[(3\theta_2 - \theta_3)/T]\left(\frac{E_2}{\theta_2 R_{CO_2}}\right)^3 (E_3 + \theta_3 R_{CO_2}) - E_3\left(\frac{E_2}{\theta_2 R_{CO_2}} + 1\right)^3\right] \\
&\quad + Z_{CN}Q\left(\overset{01}{N}, \underset{10}{C3}\right)\left[\exp[(\theta_4 - \theta_3)/T]\left(\frac{E_4}{\theta_4 R_{N_2}}\right)(E_3 + \theta_3 R_{CO_2})\right. \\
&\quad \left. - E_3\left(\frac{E_4}{\theta_4 R_{N_2}} + 1\right)\right]
\end{aligned} \tag{3.46}
$$

Note that, in Eqs. (3.44)–(3.46), the transition probabilities are a function of the gas translational (static) temperature T and can be obtained from Taylor and Bitterman (1969). Also note that the translational temperature appears explicitly in Eqs. (3.44)–(3.46) via the relationships for reverse and forward transition probabilities [see Eqs. (3.15) and (3.20)].

The vibrational rate equations for a multimode gas, of which Eqs. (3.44)–(3.46) are examples, were first addressed by Schwartz *et al.* (1952); this is the "SSH theory" often referred to in the literature. Since the advent of gasdynamic lasers in 1966, specific interest in CO_2–N_2 mixtures has resulted in several alternate derivations of the governing rate equations. Basov *et al.* (1968) quote such equations for CO_2–N_2 mixtures without derivation. In 1968, Dr. Albert Wood (presently with the Office of

Naval Research) of the Avco Everett Research Laboratory derived the rate equations for CO_2–N_2–H_2O mixtures in great detail, using the concept of "effective" relaxation times for some of the important V–V transitions; however, Wood's derivation has never been published. More recently, MacDonald (1970), in a Ph.D. thesis, derived the equations for CO_2–N_2 mixtures using kinetic rate constants rather than transition probabilities. Also, Munjee (1970, 1972) has derived the equations for a CO_2–N_2–He or H_2O mixtures. The resulting equations are quoted in Munjee (1972) without derivation; however, a development of Eq. (3.46) is given in some detail in Munjee (1970). The nomenclature and derivations in this chapter follow the work of Munjee. Indeed, the derivation in the present chapter leading to Eq. (3.44), combined with the details given in Munjee (1970) for the derivation of Eq. (3.46), provides a reasonably complete picture of the vibrational rate equations for the analysis of CO_2–N_2–H_2O or He gasdynamic lasers.

In summary, Eqs. (3.44)–(3.46) are necessary for describing the time rate of change of the nonequilibrium vibrational energies contained within the various modes of CO_2 and N_2. In these equations the transition probabilities are functions of T, and the collision frequencies $Z_{j,i}$ are functions of both pressure and temperature. Hence they are dependent on the values of the flow field variables in a gasdynamic laser. Therefore, for a calculation of gasdynamic laser performance, Eqs. (3.44)–(3.46) must be solved simultaneously with the governing flow equations of continuity, momentum, and energy. This leads directly to the subject of Chapter IV.

Chapter IV

Calculation of Gasdynamic Laser Performance

Probably the ultimate figure of merit for gasdynamic lasers is the diffraction-limited power produced per unit mass flow—the number of kilowatts per pound of gas per second. However, this figure of merit, termed the *specific power*, is the combination of both the physical properties of the laser gas as well as the optical design and overall size of the laser cavity; it is a reflection of both the physics and hardware aspects of the laser. On the other hand, small-signal gain and maximum available energy are probably better *scientific* figures of merit that indicate the quality of the laser medium itself. Therefore, in this vein, we will consider gasdynamic laser performance to encompass all three quantities—small-signal gain, maximum available power, and specific power. The purpose of this chapter is to discuss methods that allow the calculation of such quantities.

There are not many theoretical analyses available in the literature for gasdynamic laser performance. The paper by Basov *et al.* (1968) was the first major discussion of the problem for CO_2–N_2 mixtures. This was followed by Anderson (1970c) and Lee and Gowen (1971) for CO_2–N_2–H_2O and He mixtures. However, during this time, unpublished calculations were being made by engineers and scientists at Avco Everett Research Laboratory and the United Aircraft Research Laboratory. Since 1970, several additional calculations for CO_2–N_2–H_2O or He gasdynamic lasers have been published; among them are Christiansen and Tsongas (1971), Hoffman and Vlases (1972), Murty (1974), Munjee (1970, 1972), Howgate *et al.* (1972), and McLeary (1972). Each of these analyses used somewhat different numerical techniques, vibrational models, and values for the vibrational transition probabilities, rate constants, or relaxation times. This chapter will draw heavily from the approach described by Anderson (1970c), with more details contained in Anderson (1969).

4.1 Analysis of the Flow Field

The heart of a gasdynamic laser is the vibrational nonequilibrium expansion of a hot, high pressure gas through a supersonic nozzle. Therefore, in addition to the physical aspects of the molecular vibrational energy exchanges discussed in Chapter III, the flow-field properties of velocity, pressure, density, and temperature must be considered. Moreover, the flow field is fully coupled with the vibrational kinetics; i.e., the relaxation of vibrational energy described by Eqs. (3.44)–(3.46) depends in part on the flow properties, while at the same time the flow itself is influenced by the rate of energy transfer between vibration and translation. Hence the general equations that describe the conservation of mass, momentum, and total energy in the flow must be solved simultaneously with Eqs. (3.44)–(3.46). The continuity, momentum, and energy equations for a fluid flow are well known; for a high temperature gas flow, they are given in Vincenti and Kruger (1965) and Clarke and McChesney (1964). Also, for nozzle flows, it is commonplace to assume that the flow-field variables (pressure p, density ρ, velocity u, and temperature T), as well as the vibrational energies E_{12}, E_3, and E_4, vary only with longitudinal distance along the nozzle. That is, referring to Fig. 4.1, all steady flow variables depend on x. Lateral variations normal to x are assumed negligible. This assumption of

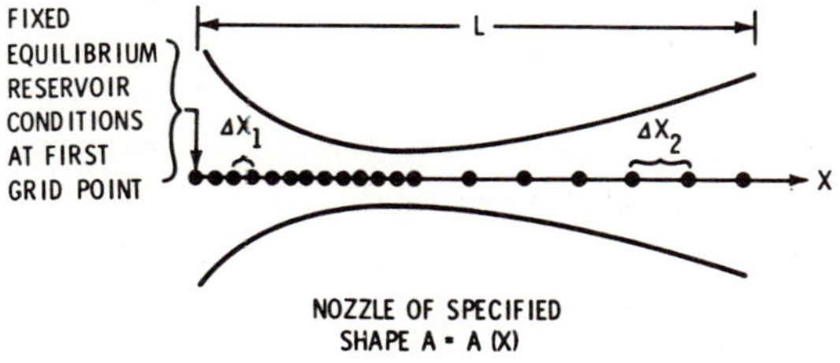

FIG. 4.1 Sketch of the coordinate system and grid points for the calculation of gasdynamic laser nozzle flows. (After Anderson, 1970c.)

a quasi-one-dimensional flow is usually sufficient for calculations of gasdynamic laser performance. As will be discussed in Chapter V, this is verified by experimental measurements of small-signal gain across the flow axis that show virtually no variation. On the other hand, the two-dimensional flow aspects dictate the *contour* (shape) of the gasdynamic laser nozzle. The contour must be determined by the two-dimensional method of characteristics, as described in any classical text on compressible flow [e.g., Liepmann and Roshko (1957) and Shapiro (1953)].

Clearly, an accurate prediction of the population inversion in an expanding gas encompasses an accurate solution of the nonequilibrium, gasdynamic flow through a convergent–divergent nozzle. Previous numerical solutions of high-temperature, quasi-one-dimensional nonequilibrium nozzle flows where vibrational and chemical nonequilibrium conditions prevail both upstream and downstream of the throat have been obtained with some effort by means of a number of independent, steadyflow analyses (Hall and Treanor, 1967). On the other hand, a useful, alternative approach has recently been presented by Anderson (1970a, d), namely, a time-dependent technique that entails the finite-difference solution of the unsteady, quasi-one-dimensional conservation equations in steps of time, starting from assumed initial distributions of the flow-field variables throughout the nozzle. The steady-state nonequilibrium nozzle flow is approached at large times. The main virtue of the time-dependent solution is its simplicity; the governing equations are solved by means of a simple, explicit, finite-difference scheme. No additional mathematical methods are necessary to treat special contingencies that can arise in the analysis of nonequilibrium nozzle flows, no difficulties are encountered in starting the nonequilibrium flow from equilibrium reservoir conditions, very large spacings can be taken between grid points along the nozzle, and the unknown critical mass flow is automatically approached at large times. As a result, no problems are encountered in the throat region with the saddle-point singularity that plagues the steady-flow formulation.

The discussion that follows is patterned after the technique described by Anderson (1970c). Consider the grid point system shown schematically in Fig. 4.1 for a nozzle of specified shape $A = A(x)$, where A is the cross-sectional area. There are two sets of equally spaced grid points. One set involves relatively fine spacing from the reservoir to slightly downstream of the throat in order to enhance numerical accuracy in the flow region where nonequilibrium phenomena develop at a fast rate, and the second set involves coarse spacing further downstream where nonequilibrium phenomena are usually progressing at a slow rate. This grid network differs from that of Anderson (1970a), which considered equally spaced grid points throughout the nozzle. In the present results 15 and 5 spaces were employed for the fine and coarse grids, respectively; i.e., a total of 21 grid points were employed throughout the nozzle.

The analysis begins by assuming initial values for the density ρ, velocity u, temperature T, and the nonequilibrium quantities q_i at all grid points throughout the nozzle. The precise quantities represented by q_i will be discussed later. Equilibrium reservoir conditions for ρ, T, and q_i are assumed at the first grid point and held fixed and invariant with time. At each internal grid point, spatial derivatives are then computed from central-finite differences,

$$\frac{\partial g}{\partial x} = \frac{g(x + \Delta x) - g(x - \Delta x)}{2\Delta x} \tag{4.1}$$

$$\frac{\partial^2 g}{\partial x^2} = \frac{g(x + \Delta x) - 2g(x) + g(x - \Delta x)}{(\Delta x)^2} \tag{4.2}$$

where g stands for ρ, u, T, and q_i. The numbers for the x-derivatives obtained from Eqs. (4.1) and (4.2) are then substituted into the quasi-one-dimensional, unsteady, conservation equations

Continuity

$$\frac{\partial \rho}{\partial t} = -\frac{1}{A}\frac{\partial(\rho u A)}{\partial x} \tag{4.3}$$

Momentum

$$\frac{\partial u}{\partial t} = -\left[\frac{1}{\rho}\frac{\partial p}{\partial x} + u\frac{\partial u}{\partial x}\right] \tag{4.4}$$

Energy

$$\frac{\partial e}{\partial t} = -\left[\frac{p}{\rho}\left(\frac{\partial u}{\partial x} + u\frac{\partial \ln A}{\partial x}\right) + u\frac{\partial e}{\partial x}\right] \tag{4.5}$$

Rate

$$\frac{\partial q_i}{\partial t} = \dot{w}_i(\rho, T, q_i) - u\frac{\partial q_i}{\partial x} \tag{4.6}$$

State

$$p = \rho R T \tag{4.7}$$

where q_i can be the population or energy per unit mass associated with a given vibrational energy level (or grouping of levels), and $\dot{w}_i$ is the net internal rate of production of q_i due to detailed vibration–vibration and vibration–translation collisions within the gas mixture. For the detailed kinetic model discussed in Chapter III, q_i in Eq. (4.6) is alternately E_{12}, E_3, and E_4, and $\dot{w}_i$ is identically equal to Eqs. (3.44)–(3.46). [Strictly speaking, q_i in Eq. (4.6) should be taken per unit mass of mixture; i.e., q_i should be alternately $c_{CO_2}E_{12}$, $c_{CO_2}E_3$, and $c_{N_2}E_4$, where c_i is the mass fraction of species i. However, for a mixture in which the chemical composition is fixed, such as in the nozzle and cavity flow of a gasdynamic laser, the mass fractions are constant and cancel in Eq. (4.6). This would not be the case for a chemically reacting gas.]

Values of the time derivatives $\partial g/\partial t$ are directly obtained from Eqs. (4.3) through (4.7), and these numbers are subsequently inserted into an expression containing the first three terms of a Taylor's series expansion in time; i.e.,

$$g(t + \Delta t) = g(t) + (\partial g/\partial t)_t \Delta t + (\partial^2 g/\partial t^2)_t (\Delta t^2/2) \tag{4.8}$$

Equation (4.8) allows the direct computation of all flow-field variables at all internal grid points at time $(t + \Delta t)$ from the known flow-field variables at time t. Values for $g(t)$ are known; as previously noted, values for $(\partial g/\partial t)_t$ are obtained from Eqs. (4.3) through (4.7). Numbers for $(\partial^2 g/\partial t^2)_t$ can be obtained by differentiation of Eqs. (4.3) through (4.6) with respect to t. However, such an operation introduces mixed derivatives $\partial^2 g/\partial x\, \partial t$, values for which are simply obtained by differentiation of Eqs. (4.3) through (4.6) with respect to x. Hence, starting from assumed initial values for the flow-field variables throughout the nozzle, new values of the flow-field distributions are computed in steps of time from Eq. (4.8), continuing for many time steps until the steady-state solution is approached at large times (where $\partial g/\partial t$ and $\partial^2 g/\partial t^2$ both approach zero). For the present study, this steady-state solution is the desired result.

The most recent calculations using the above approach employ a slightly modified technique discussed by Anderson (1970b, d). The modification consists of using

$$g(t + \Delta t) = g(t) + (\partial g/\partial t)_{av} \Delta t \tag{4.9}$$

in lieu of Eq. (4.8). Here, the time derivative is not evaluated at time t as in Eq. (4.8); rather, an average value between t and $(t + \Delta t)$ is utilized. This average value is obtained from the general method of MacCormack (1969), who has shown that the general scheme is of second-order accuracy. The results obtained are the same using either approach. However, by using Eq. (4.9) with MacCormack's finite-difference scheme, a considerable simplification in computer programming and reductions in execution time are obtained. See Anderson (1970d) for more details.

The value of Δt employed in Eqs. (4.8) and (4.9) must satisfy two stability criteria:

$$\Delta t \leq \Delta x/(u + a) \tag{4.10}$$

where a is the local frozen speed of sound, and

$$\Delta t < \tau \tag{4.11}$$

where τ is the characteristic relaxation time for the fastest finite-rate molecular relaxation process occurring within the mixture. Equation (4.10) is the Courant–Friedrichs–Levy (1928) stability criterion, which, in physical terms, states that Δt must be no greater than the time required for a sound wave to propagate from one grid point to the next; and Eq. (4.11) states that Δt must be no greater than the characteristic time of the finite-rate molecular energy exchange processes occurring within the flowing gas. This latter stability criterion is plausible on physical grounds and has been demonstrated empirically by Anderson (1970a).

Because central finite-differences are employed, Eqs. (4.1) through (4.9) can be applied to the internal points only. For each time step, values for ρ, u, T, and q_i at the last grid point (nozzle exit) and u at the first grid point (nozzle inlet) are obtained by extrapolation, as discussed by Anderson (1970a). Also, for the actual numerical computations, Eqs. (4.1) through (4.11) are rewritten in nondimensional form so that the magnitudes of all variables are of order unity or smaller.

4.2 Vibrational Model

The vibrational energy level diagram for CO_2 and N_2 is once again shown in Fig. 4.2; however, Fig. 4.2 goes one step further than Fig. 3.4. As discussed in Chapter III, the Fermi resonance between the (100) and (020) levels in CO_2 leads to the assumption of local equilibrium between the ν_1 and ν_2 modes. This is illustrated by the box shown in Figure 3.4. Now, in addition, we consider the fact that the (001) level of CO_2 and the $v = 1$ level of N_2 differ by only 18 cm^{-1}; hence these two levels are in close resonance. As a result, if there are no strong radiative effects (no laser power extraction), the ν_3 mode of CO_2 and the N_2 may also be assumed to be in local equilibrium. This assumption is reasonable for calculations of small-signal gain and maximum available energy where radiative effects are indeed negligible; however, it is *not* valid for calculations of power extraction, as will be discussed later.

Therefore, in Fig. 4.2, the ν_1 and ν_2 modes are grouped together in a box

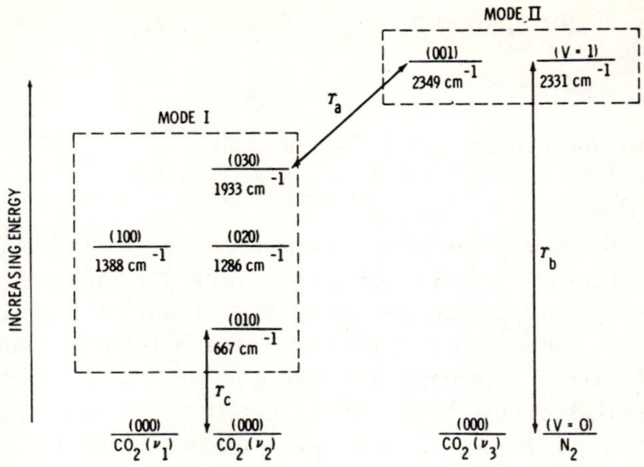

FIG. 4.2 A simplified vibrational kinetic model for CO_2–N_2. (After Anderson, 1970c.)

labeled Mode I, and the ν_3 mode and N_2 are grouped together in another box labeled Mode II. These modes are assumed to be in equilibrium within themselves, but not with each other nor with the translational mode. This leads to a "three temperature model": the vibrational temperatures of Modes I and II, $T_{\mathrm{vib_I}}$ and $T_{\mathrm{vib_{II}}}$, respectively, and the translational temperature T of the gas. The net effect of all the complex vibrational energy exchanges taking place due to molecular collisions now reduces to the relaxation of Mode II via τ_a and τ_b and the relaxation of Mode I, principally via τ_c. The relaxation times τ_a, τ_b, and τ_c are shown in Fig. 4.2 and are discussed in subsequent paragraphs. For typical gasdynamic laser conditions, $\tau_b : \tau_a : \tau_c$ are crudely in the ratio 100 : 10 : 1. Indeed, the N_2 vibrational energy relaxes very slowly under a sudden change in temperature. In fact, pure N_2 has the longest relaxation time of any diatomic molecule known to the author. Since the $v = 1$ level of N_2 is closely coupled to the CO_2 (001) level, the entire Mode II relaxes slowly. On the other hand, τ_c is generally quite small; hence, Mode I (the ν_1 and ν_2 modes) equilibrates very rapidly with changes in temperature.

Now we can see in a qualitative sense how the inversion occurs in a supersonic expansion. In the reservoir we have a hot, vibrationally excited mixture of CO_2–N_2–H_2O or He. Molecules are populating the higher lying energy levels, but, since the gas is in thermal equilibrium in the reservoir, there are fewer molecules in (001) than there are in (100). When the gas expands through the supersonic nozzle, the temperature drops dramatically. In the process Mode II relaxes slowly, whereas Mode I relaxes rapidly.

Molecules slowly drop out of the (001) level and rapidly drop out of the (100) level. In other words the population of the (001) level, N_{001}, tends to "hang up" or "freeze," whereas the population of the (100) level is rapidly depleted due to the fast equilibration with the cooled gas. The net result can be a population inversion, i.e., $N_{001} > N_{100}$. A major role of H_2O or He in this scheme, as we understand it at present, is to speed up the equilibration of Mode I, hence increasing the population inversion.

In the following discussion of the vibrational model, a CO_2–N_2–H_2O mixture will be assumed for purposes of illustration. CO_2–N_2–He is handled in the same manner, with H_2O replaced by He in all subsequent equations.

The net vibrational energies per unit mass contained within each "mode," $(e_{\text{vib}})_{\text{I}}$ and $(e_{\text{vib}})_{\text{II}}$, are chosen as the dependent nonequilibrium variables; hence Eq. (4.6) represents two rate equations with $q_i = (e_{\text{vib}})_{\text{I}}$ and $(e_{\text{vib}})_{\text{II}}$, respectively. The relaxation of these energies is assumed to be described by the simple harmonic oscillator relaxation equations

$$\dot{w}_i = \frac{d(e_{\text{vib}})_{\text{I}}}{dt} = \frac{1}{\tau_{\text{I}}}[(e_{\text{vib}})_{\text{I}}^{\text{eq}} - (e_{\text{vib}})_{\text{I}}] \tag{4.12a}$$

when $q_i = (e_{\text{vib}})_{\text{I}}$ and

$$\dot{w}_i = \frac{d(e_{\text{vib}})_{\text{II}}}{dt} = \frac{1}{\tau_{\text{II}}}[(e_{\text{vib}})_{\text{II}}^{\text{eq}} - (e_{\text{vib}})_{\text{II}}] \tag{4.12b}$$

when $q_i = (e_{\text{vib}})_{\text{II}}$. In Eqs. (4.12a) and (4.12b), $(e_{\text{vib}})_{\text{I}}^{\text{eq}}$ and $(e_{\text{vib}})_{\text{II}}^{\text{eq}}$ are the equilibrium vibrational energies that would be contained in Modes I and II, respectively, at the local gas translational temperature T, and τ_{I} and τ_{II} are the characteristic relaxation times for Modes I and II, respectively. τ_{I} and τ_{II} are averages that characterize the net rate of energy transfer into and out of Modes I and II; this energy transfer is assumed to be governed by the major transitions (heavy arrows in Fig. 4.2), which are identified with the relaxation times τ_{a}, τ_{b}, τ_{c}. These relaxation times are themselves averages of the detailed CO_2–CO_2, CO_2–N_2, CO_2–H_2O, N_2–N_2, and N_2–H_2O collisions. Such averages for a mixture of gases are obtained from the "parallel resistance" mixture rule

$$\frac{1}{\tau_{\text{a}}} = \frac{X_{CO_2}}{(\tau_{\text{a}})_{CO_2-CO_2}} + \frac{X_{N_2}}{(\tau_{\text{a}})_{CO_2-N_2}} + \frac{X_{H_2O}}{(\tau_{\text{a}})_{CO_2-H_2O}} \tag{4.13a}$$

$$\frac{1}{\tau_{\text{b}}} = \frac{X_{CO_2}}{(\tau_{\text{b}})_{N_2-CO_2}} + \frac{X_{N_2}}{(\tau_{\text{b}})_{N_2-N_2}} + \frac{X_{H_2O}}{(\tau_{\text{b}})_{N_2-H_2O}} \tag{4.13b}$$

$$\frac{1}{\tau_{\text{c}}} = \frac{X_{CO_2}}{(\tau_{\text{c}})_{CO_2-CO_2}} + \frac{X_{N_2}}{(\tau_{\text{c}})_{CO_2-N_2}} + \frac{X_{H_2O}}{(\tau_{\text{c}})_{CO_2-H_2O}} \tag{4.13c}$$

where X_i denotes the mole fraction of chemical species i. For the present results, values for the denominators of the terms on the right-hand side of Eqs. (4.13a, b, and c) are obtained directly from Taylor and Bitterman (1967). (However, the reader should consult Appendixes A and B for more recent kinetic rates.) In turn, the average relaxation times for Modes I and II are obtained from

$$\tau_{\mathrm{I}} = \tau_{\mathrm{C}} \tag{4.14}$$

$$\frac{1}{\tau_{\mathrm{II}}} = \left[\frac{X_{\mathrm{CO_2}}}{\tau_{\mathrm{a}}} + \frac{X_{\mathrm{N_2}}}{\tau_{\mathrm{b}}}\right] \frac{1}{(X_{\mathrm{CO_2}} + X_{\mathrm{N_2}})} \tag{4.15}$$

These values are subsequently employed in equations (4.12a and b).

Parenthetically, the general quantity τ can be interpreted as a mean time required for a single particle to make a transition from one state to another state due to collisions with other particles. In turn, τ^{-1} can be interpreted as the number of transitions per second per particle. Hence, on a physical basis, Eqs. (4.13a, b, and c) simply state that the total number of transitions per second per particle due to collisions with all species present in the mixture is the sum of the transitions per second per particle due to collisions with each individual species. Equations (4.14) and (4.15) have similar physical interpretations, except now the "transitions" are from one mode to another.

The above model for treating the complex vibrational energy transfer processes is approximate, firstly because of the use of Modes I and II shown in Fig. 4.2, and secondly because of the simplified rate equations given by Eqs. (4.12a and b). The form of Eqs. (4.12a and b) is exact only for a diatomic simple harmonic oscillator. We have derived much more detailed and exact rate equations for the CO_2–N_2 system in Chapter III. By comparison, Eqs. (4.12a and b) are linear equations that only approximate the more exact Eqs. (3.44)–(3.46). However, Eqs. (4.12a and b) are simpler to apply, and they yield results that are in reasonable agreement with results obtained with more detailed models and with experimental data (see Chapter V). This simplified model has been employed by Anderson (1970c) and Lee and Gowen (1971), whereas more detailed models represented by Eqs. (3.44)–(3.46) have been employed by Basov *et al.* (1968), Munjee (1972), and MacDonald (1970). Again we emphasize that the simplified model represented by Modes I and II in Fig. 4.2 and by Eqs. (4.12a)–(4.15) is intended only for the calculation of population inversions in CO_2–N_2–H_2O or He mixtures; it is not necessarily valid for other gases, nor can it be used when substantial amounts of radiative energy interact with the gas.

Referring again to Eqs. (4.12a) and (4.12b), $(e_{\mathrm{vib}})_{\mathrm{I}}$ and $(e_{\mathrm{vib}})_{\mathrm{II}}$ are treated as the dependent nonequilibrium variables. From these energies different vibrational temperatures, T_{vib_I} and T_{vib_II}, are defined from the following equilibrium relations [based on the results from Chapter III, such as Eq. (3.4)].

$$(e_{\text{vib}})_\text{I} = c_{CO_2} R_{CO_2} \left\{ \left(\frac{h\nu_1}{k}\right) [\exp(h\nu_1/kT_{\text{vib}_\text{I}}) - 1]^{-1} + (2h\nu_2/k)[\exp(h\nu_2/kT_{\text{vib}_\text{I}}) - 1]^{-1} \right\} \tag{4.16a}$$

and

$$(e_{\text{vib}})_\text{II} = c_{CO_2} R_{CO_2} \left(\frac{h\nu_3}{k}\right) [\exp(h\nu_3/kT_{\text{vib}_\text{II}}) - 1]^{-1} + c_{N_2} R_{N_2} \left(\frac{h\nu}{k}\right) [\exp(h\nu/kT_{\text{vib}_\text{II}}) - 1]^{-1} \tag{4.16b}$$

In Eqs. (4.16a and b) c_{CO_2} and R_{CO_2} are the mass fraction and specific gas constant, respectively, for CO_2; c_{N_2} and R_{N_2} are defined similarly for N_2; ν_1, ν_2, and ν_3 are the normal vibrational frequencies of the symmetric stretching, the bending, and the asymmetric stretching modes, respectively, for CO_2; and ν is the normal vibrational frequency for N_2. In turn T_{vib_I} and T_{vib_II} are used to compute populations of energy levels within Modes I and II, assuming a Boltzmann distribution locally within each mode. For example, the population of the (001) level in CO_2 is obtained from

$$N_{001} = N_{CO_2} \exp(-h\nu_3/kT_{\text{vib}_\text{II}})/Q \tag{4.17}$$

where

$$Q = [1 - \exp(-h\nu_1/kT_{\text{vib}_\text{I}})]^{-1}[1 - \exp(-h\nu_2/kT_{\text{vib}_\text{I}})]^{-2} \times [1 - \exp(-h\nu_3/kT_{\text{vib}_\text{II}})]^{-1} \tag{4.18}$$

and the population of the (100) level in CO_2 is obtained from

$$N_{100} = N_{CO_2} \exp(-h\nu_1/kT_{\text{vib}_\text{I}})/Q \tag{4.19}$$

In the above formulation, the role of H_2O or He as a catalyst enters the analysis through its presence in Eqs. (4.13a, b, and c).

As a final note with regard to the present analysis, $(e_{\text{vib}})_\text{I}$ and $(e_{\text{vib}})_\text{II}$ are inherent parts of the time-dependent nonequilibrium nozzle flow solution and are computed at each time step during the transient approach to steady-state conditions. Then, after the steady state is achieved, the vibrational temperatures and populations are computed from Eqs. (4.16a) through (4.19).

4.3 Results

The numerical nature of the time-dependent, vibrational nonequilibrium nozzle solution is clearly shown in Fig. 4.3, which illustrates the shape of the $(e_{vib})_{II}$ distribution through a wedge nozzle at several times during its approach to the steady state. In Fig. 4.3, R is the specific gas constant for the mixture. The dotted line shows the assumed initial distribution at $t = 0$, the solid lines show distributions after 400, 800, and 1000 time steps,

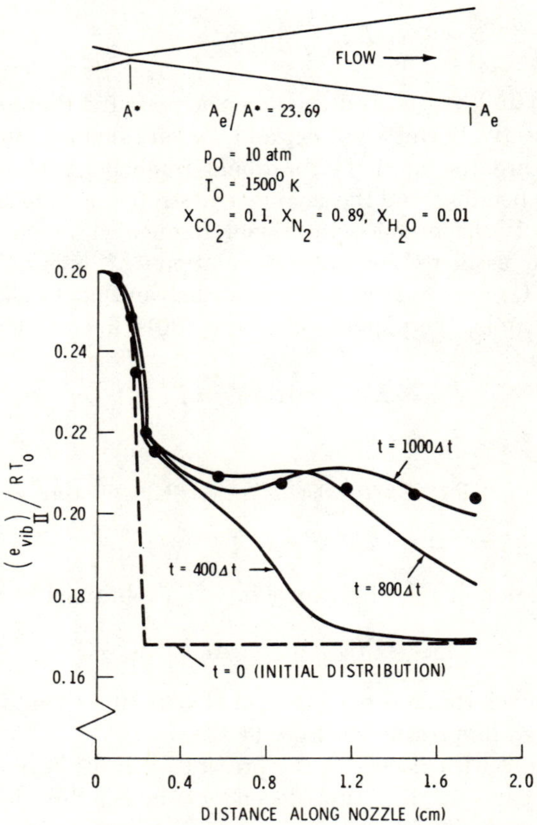

FIG. 4.3 Distribution of transient and final steady-state (●, $t = 3000\ \Delta t$) Mode II vibrational energy along the nozzle.

and the solid dots show the final, steady-state, nonequilibrium distribution obtained after approximately 3000 time steps. Similar transient variations and the subsequent approach to the steady state occur for all other flow variables throughout the nozzle.

The final, steady-state $(e_{vib})_{II}$ distribution shown in Fig. 4.3, taken in conjunction with the simultaneous steady-state $(e_{vib})_{I}$ distribution, leads to the steady-flow results shown in Figs. 4.4 through 4.6. In Fig. 4.4, the two vibrational temperature distributions are compared with the translational temperature distribution. Note that Mode II relaxes much slower than Mode I and that both Modes I and II are not in equilibrium with the local translational temperature except near the nozzle reservoir. Note also that $(T_{vib})_{II}$ begins to diverge from T in the subsonic section of the nozzle, with $[(T_{vib})_{II} - T] = 120°K$ at the throat. Hence nonequilibrium effects upstream of the throat are noticeable. In Fig. 4.5, the populations N_{001} and N_{100} of the (001) and (100) levels, respectively, in CO_2 are shown as functions of distance along the wedge nozzle. At approximately 0.26 cm downstream of the throat, the populations of the (001) and (100) levels are equal, and a substantial population inversion develops further downstream. This population inversion is shown in Fig. 4.6 in terms of $(N_{001} - N_{100})/N_{CO_2}$, where N_{CO_2} is the local number density

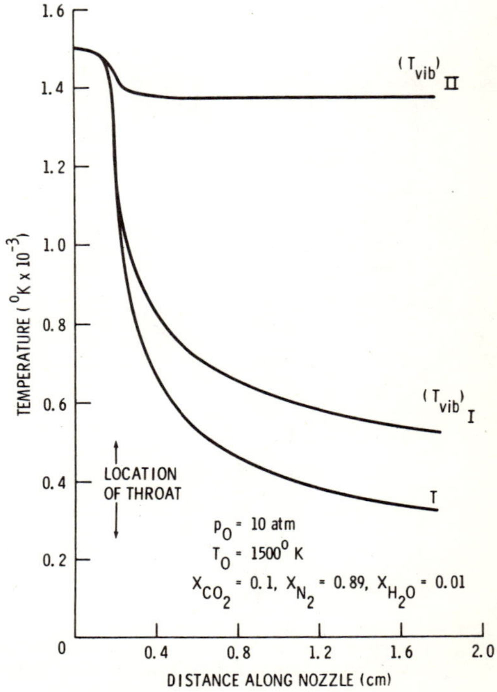

FIG. 4.4 Comparison of the steady-state vibrational and translational temperature distributions throughout the nozzle.

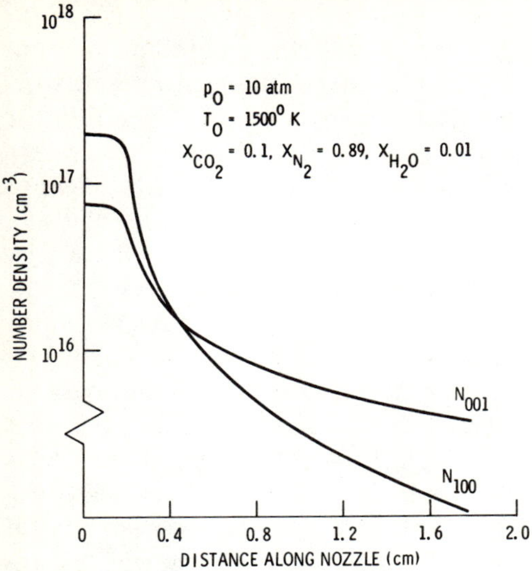

FIG. 4.5 Steady-state population distributions through the nozzle.

of CO_2 particles. If the nozzle exhausts into a constant area duct as shown in Fig. 4.6, the inversion will continue to increase beyond the nozzle exit until Mode I equilibrates with T, beyond which the inversion will slowly decrease due to the moderate deactivation of Mode II. As emphasized

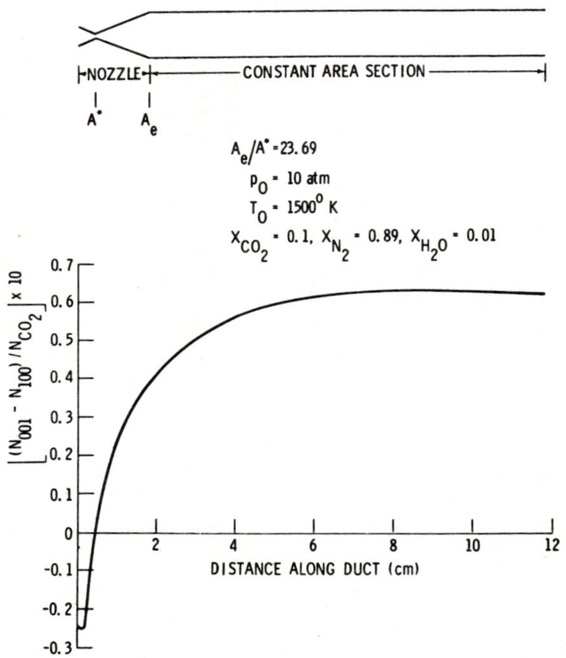

FIG. 4.6 Steady-state distribution of population inversion through the nozzle.

by Taylor and Bitterman (1969) and Anderson and Harris (1972a), the equilibration of Mode I with T is enhanced by the presence of H_2O in the mixture.

4.4 Comparison with Basov

Basov *et al.* (1968) have published results for population inversions created in a supersonic expansion of a CO_2–N_2 mixture through a hyperbolic nozzle. In contrast to the present results, shown in Figs. 4.3 through 4.6, Basov did not include the effect of H_2O on the population inversions. Also in contrast to the present analysis, Basov assumed equilibrium conditions from the reservoir to the throat. In order to provide a comparison with the results of Basov *et al.* (1968), results are obtained with the present time-dependent analysis for a nozzle shape, p_0, T_0, and mixture ratio indentical to those of Basov *et al.* (1968). Figures 4.7 and 4.8 show the resulting

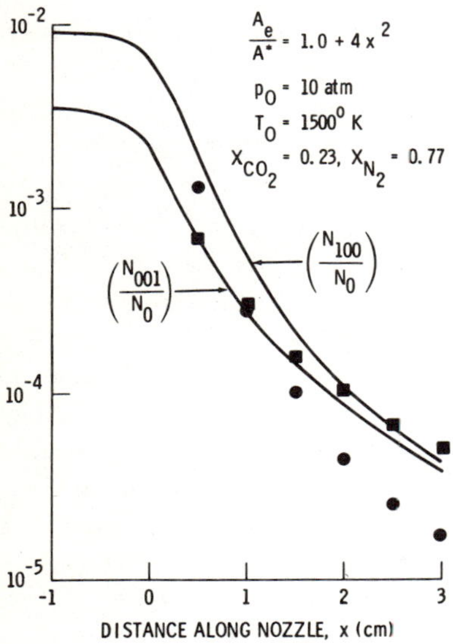

FIG. 4.7

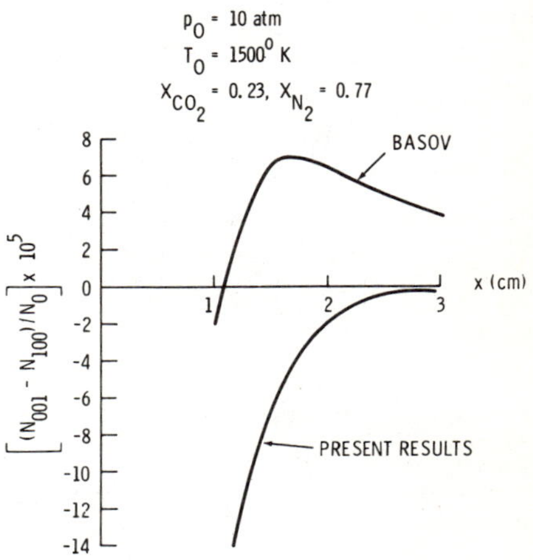

FIG. 4.8

FIG. 4.7 Steady-state population distributions through the nozzle; comparison of time-dependent calculations of Anderson (1970c)(—)with those of Basov *et al.* (1968) (●, ■).

FIG. 4.8 Steady-state distribution of population inversion through the nozzle; comparison of time-dependent calculations of Anderson (1970c) with those of Basov *et al.* (1968).

comparison. Figure 4.7 illustrates the populations N_{100} and N_{001} as a function of distance through the nozzle, and Fig. 4.8 shows the population inversion distribution throughout the nozzle. N_0 is the total reservoir number density for the gas mixture. A study of Fig. 4.7 shows that Basov predicts a slower relaxation of the (001) level and a faster relaxation of the (100) level in comparion with the present results. Consequently, as seen in Fig. 4.8, Basov's results show a population inversion, whereas, for the given conditions, the present results predict no population inversion. The present results embody detailed information on transition probabilities reported by Taylor and Bitterman (1967), whereas Basov used somewhat cruder information for transition probabilities. A comparison of these two sets of transition data show approximate agreement for the collision probability for deactivation of the (001) level. On the other hand, Basov used probabilities for deactivation of the (010) level [hence the (100) level, which is closely coupled by fast resonant exchanges] that are more than an order of magnitude larger than those presented by Taylor and Bitterman (1967). Consequently, the differences shown in Figs. 4.7 and 4.8 can be attributed mainly to differences in relaxation times used for the two analyses. Taylor's and Bitterman's thorough compilation of transition probabilities is believed to contain the most reliable data currently available in the literature. These data have been very recently updated by Anderson (1973, 1974). (See Appendixes A and B of the present book.) These results also clearly demonstrate that population inversions in CO_2–N_2 mixtures *without* a catalyst are difficult to obtain. Indeed, in subsequent sections of this book we will see that the presence of H_2O or He is vitally necessary for the attainment of reasonable population inversions.

As a point of interest, Basov's assumption of equilibrium conditions at the nozzle throat is reasonable for the nozzle shape he considered; for this nozzle, the subsonic approach to the throat is relatively long and smooth, thus enhancing equilibrium conditions. In fact, the present results, which include nonequilibrium conditions upstream of the throat, indicate that $[(T_{\text{vib}})_{\text{II}} - T]$ is 28°K at the throat for Basov's conditions. This should be compared with the 120°K difference obtained for the shorter nozzle considered in Fig. 4.3, where nonequilibrium effects upstream of the throat are considerable.

4.5 Coupled and Uncoupled Flows

With regard to calculations of population inversions in an expanding nozzle flow, there has been some question concerning the error induced by uncoupling the gasdynamic flow-field from the vibrational relaxation phenomena. For example, the calculation of population inversions would be greatly simplified if the pressure, temperature, and velocity distributions were obtained from a calculation of frozen or equilibrium nozzle flows and then used to solve independently the vibrational rate equations. The flow variable most severely affected by these uncoupled solutions is translational (static) temperature. Since the relaxation rates depend exponentially on T, and because N_{100} tries to equilibrate with T in the supersonic stream, the theoretical population inversions obtained from such uncoupled solutions may contain an inordinate error.

In order to examine this question, a numerical experiment is performed using the present time-dependent analysis to compute population in-

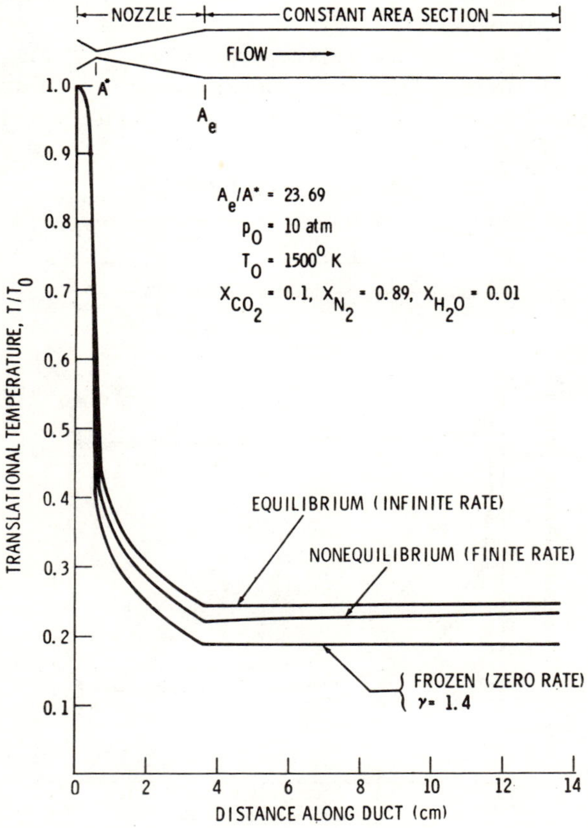

FIG. 4.9 Comparison of steady-state temperature distributions for equilibrium, frozen, and finite-rate nozzle flow.

versions for the following cases: (1) Coupled, where the finite-rate, vibrational energy relaxation is fully included in the gasdynamic energy equation; (2) uncoupled (equilibrium), where p, T, and u are obtained from an expansion assuming infinite-rate, vibrational equilibrium; and (3) uncoupled (frozen), where p, T, and u are obtained from an expansion assuming a zero vibrational rate, i.e., frozen flow. In case (3) two sets of results are obtained, where the ratio of specific heats γ equals 1.4 and 1.3. The value of 1.4 properly corresponds to a vibrationally frozen expansion of CO_2 and N_2, whereas the value of 1.3 is of interest only because it is equal to the equilibrium value of the ratio of specific heats for the gas mixture in the reservoir. For all of the above cases, a simple wedge nozzle followed by a constant area duct was assumed. This geometry and the reservoir conditions are described in Fig. 4.9. Note that this nozzle has the same area ratio but twice the length of the wedge nozzle previously considered in Figs. 4.3 through 4.6.

Results from this numerical experiment are shown in Fig. 4.9 through 4.12. Figure 4.9 contrasts the translational temperature distributions obtained for the different assumptions of infinite, finite, and frozen rates.

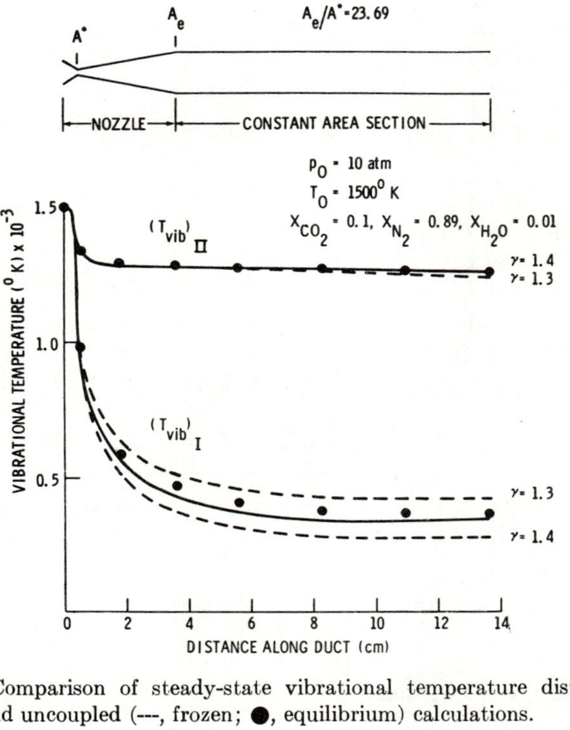

FIG. 4.10 Comparison of steady-state vibrational temperature distributions for coupled (—) and uncoupled (---, frozen; ●, equilibrium) calculations.

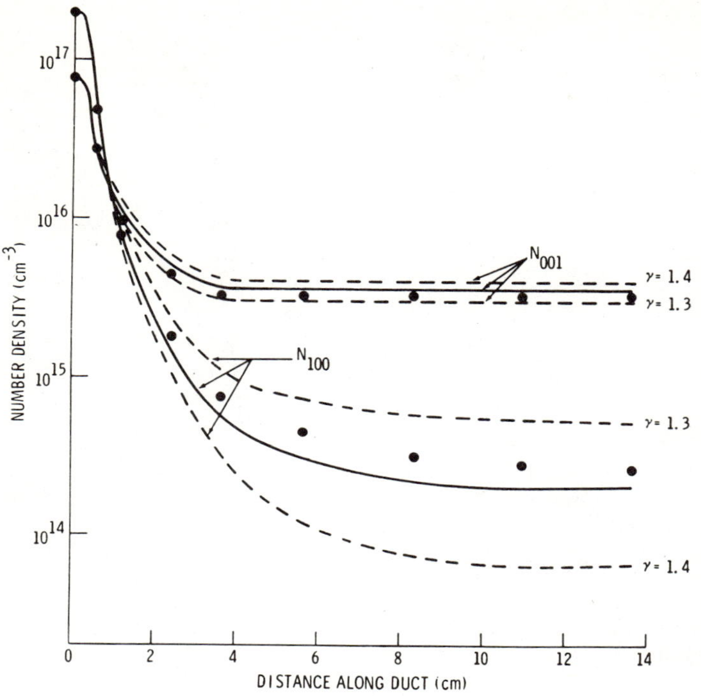

FIG. 4.11 Comparison of steady-state number density distributions for coupled (—) and uncoupled (---, frozen; ●, equilibrium) calculations.

Such a comparison is classical and is presented in order to help interpret the subsequent results. Figure 4.9 also shows that, for the present conditions, the actual nonequilibrium expansion is closer to equilibrium than frozen. In turn, a comparison of the curves shown in Fig. 4.10 indicates that $(T_{vib})_I$ is more strongly affected than $(T_{vib})_{II}$. Indeed, the upper level appears to be insensitive to the differences in translational temperature between the different cases despite the exponential variation of relaxation time with T. The reason for the differences in $(T_{vib})_I$ is the strong tendency of the lower level to equilibrate with T, which is different for each of the cases.

The differences in $(T_{vib})_I$ shown in Fig. 4.10 are magnified when N_{100} is computed, as shown in Fig. 4.11. Also, as expected from the very small differences in $(T_{vib})_{II}$, only small differences occur in N_{001}.

The differences shown in Fig. 4.11 translate into the differences in population inversion shown in Fig. 4.12. Among the simplified, uncoupled cases, Fig. 4.12 illustrates that the p, T, and u variations obtained from an

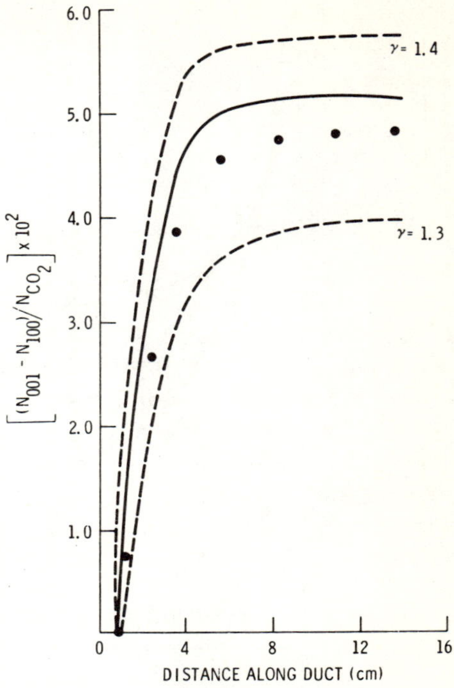

FIG. 4.12 Comparison of steady-state population inversion distributions for coupled (—) and uncoupled (---, frozen; ●, equilibrium) calculations.

equilibrium flow calculation provide the closest comparison with the coupled case. However, there is still a noticeable error induced by all the uncoupled cases. With regard to the frozen cases, one might be able to simulate the coupled results by "proper" choice of an effective γ between 1.3 and 1.4. However, such a value of γ is not known a priori, and its proper choice would be strictly fortuitous without first knowing the answer.

Reflecting upon the results shown in Figs. 4.9 through 4.12, the accurate calculation of population inversions in an expanding gas apparently requires an analysis that fully takes into account the coupling between the finite-rate nonequilibrium processes and the gasdynamic flow.

It is interesting to note that, for the same reservoir conditions, the peak population inversion shown in Fig. 4.6 is 23% higher than the peak shown in Fig. 4.12 for the coupled case. The larger inversion shown in Fig. 4.6 is due solely to the shorter nozzle length and is to be expected due to a greater degree of nonequilibrium in the shorter nozzle flow.

4.6 Recapitulation

The previous sections have described the time-dependent technique for calculating population inversions in an expanding gas and have given some typical results obtained with an approximate vibrational model. The kinetic rates employed in generating the results shown in Figs. 4.3 through 4.12 are given in Appendix A of Anderson (1969), which contains simple correlations of the rates from Taylor and Bitterman (1967). However, these correlations have been improved, as discussed by Anderson (1973, 1974), and the reader is again urged to consult Appendixes A and B of the present book for updated kinetic rates.

Another detailed numerical solution for GDLs (gasdynamic lasers) was obtained by Munjee (1972), who incorporated a more detailed kinetic model than that used by Anderson (1970c). Munjee's kinetic model is patterned after that of Basov *et al.* (1968); however, unlike Basov, Munjee includes the effect of a catalyst (H_2O or He) in the master rate equations. Munjee's work serves as the basis for the theoretical results quoted by Christiansen and Tsongas (1971) and Buonadonna and Christiansen (1973). In addition to these detailed numerical solutions, a useful approximate analysis has been developed by Hoffman and Vlases (1972). Recent results using the sudden-freezing approximation have also been reported by Murty (1974).

4.7 Power Extraction

In a gasdynamic laser, the energy available for laser power extraction is contained in the vibrational energies of the excited N_2 and $CO_2(\nu_3)$ at the exit of the supersonic nozzle. The challenge is to optically extract as much of this available energy as possible before it deactivates and "leaks" into translational and rotational energy due to molecular collisions. Moreover, the extraction process should also produce a good quality, near-diffraction-limited beam. Therefore, the optical design of the laser cavity is of utmost importance. Some considerations dealing with the optical cavity will be discussed in Chapter X, and some of the aerodynamic disturbances that influence cavity design and beam quality will also be treated in Chapter X. However, let us now consider power extraction from a purely energy standpoint.

The *maximum available laser energy* can be calculated as follows. Consider a point in the nozzle of a gasdynamic laser. Using the notation of Anderson (1970c), the translational and rotational temperature at this point is T, the sum of the vibrational energy contained in the excited N_2 and CO_2 (ν_3) is $e_{\text{vib}_{\text{II}}}$ with an attendant vibrational temperature $T_{\text{vib}_{\text{II}}}$, the sum of the vibrational energy in the $CO_2(\nu_1)$ and $CO_2(\nu_2)$ modes is $e_{\text{vib}_{\text{I}}}$ with an attendant $T_{\text{vib}_{\text{I}}}$, and the population densities of the upper and lower laser levels are N_{001} and N_{100}, respectively. In GDL flows in general, $T_{\text{vib}_{\text{II}}} > T_{\text{vib}_{\text{I}}} > T$. When an inversion exists, then, by definition, $N_{001} - N_{100} > 0$. The population densities are given by

$$N_{001} = (N_{CO_2}/Q) \exp(-\epsilon_{001}/kT_{\text{vib}_{\text{II}}})$$

$$N_{100} = (N_{CO_2}/Q) \exp(-\epsilon_{100}/kT_{\text{vib}_{\text{I}}})$$

where Q is the partition function. We ask the following question: If energy is drained from $e_{\text{vib}_{\text{II}}}$ and $e_{\text{vib}_{\text{I}}}$ is held constant, at what value of $T_{\text{vib}_{\text{II}}}$ will the population inversion go to zero? Denote this value of $T_{\text{vib}_{\text{II}}}$ by $(T_{\text{vib}_{\text{II}}}{}^{\circ})$. Then,

$$N_{001} - N_{100} = 0 = (N_{CO_2}/Q)[\exp(-\epsilon_{001}/k(T_{\text{vib}_{\text{II}}}{}^{\circ})) - \exp(-\epsilon_{100}/kT_{\text{vib}_{\text{I}}})]$$

Hence,

$$\epsilon_{001}/k(T_{\text{vib}_{\text{II}}}{}^{\circ}) = \epsilon_{100}/kT_{\text{vib}_{\text{I}}}$$

Thus,

$$(T_{\text{vib}_{\text{II}}}{}^{\circ}) = T_{\text{vib}_{\text{I}}}(\epsilon_{001}/\epsilon_{100})$$

When $T_{\text{vib}_{\text{II}}} > (T_{\text{vib}_{\text{II}}}{}^{\circ})$, an inversion exists and laser power can in principle be extracted. When $T_{\text{vib}_{\text{II}}} < (T_{\text{vib}_{\text{II}}}{}^{\circ})$, no inversion is present and no power can be extracted.

In order to consider the maximum laser energy available, we assume that $T_{\text{vib}_{\text{I}}} = T$. Then, $(T_{\text{vib}_{\text{II}}}{}^{\circ}) = T(\epsilon_{001}/\epsilon_{100})$. Using this value of $(T_{\text{vib}_{\text{II}}}{}^{\circ})$, we define a maximum available laser energy as

$$e_{\max} = 0.409[e_{\text{vib}_{\text{II}}}(T_{\text{vib}_{\text{II}}}) - e_{\text{vib}_{\text{II}}}(T_{\text{vib}_{\text{II}}}{}^{\circ})]$$

where the factor 0.409 is the quantum efficiency for the CO_2 laser transition at 10.6 μm.

The quantity $e_{\max}$ is a convenient index to gauge the amount of power that might be extracted from a gasdynamic laser. However, in reality the actual power extraction is usually less than $e_{\max}$ due to losses in the laser cavity. Also, all values of $e_{\max}$ given in the present book are local values at the nozzle exit, where $T_{\text{vib}_{\text{II}}}$ is obtained from the coupled analysis of Anderson (1970c). Therefore, the present values of $e_{\max}$ account for the kinetic deactivation losses in the nozzle. This is in contrast to previously simpler but less realistic definitions of maximum available power (Gerry, 1970), which have been based strictly on the vibrational energy in the reservoir.

We emphasize again that $e_{\max}$ is simply a convenient index that represents an upper limit and that the actual power extracted may be quite different. An accurate calculation of power extraction must combine a detailed numerical solution of the nonequilibrium supersonic flow in the cavity coupled with a point-by-point numerical integration of the radiative transfer equation

$$dI_\nu/I_\nu = G\,dy \tag{4.20}$$

in a direction normal to the flow. Here, G is the actual gain (proportional to the actual population inversion) that takes into account the local depopulation of the N_2 and CO_2 (ν_3) levels and the population of the CO_2 (ν_1) levels due to interaction with the laser radiation. G is less than G_0, which is the small-signal gain coefficient discussed previously. This calculation should be at least a "two-dimensional" analysis, where I_ν varies in the flow direction as well as in the beam direction perpendicular to the flow. Such detailed calculations have been performed by Gerhard Heiche and E. L. Harris at the Naval Ordnance Laboratory (NOL), but they are not generally available in the literature. However, for the sake of comparison, the following example is given to compare e_{max} with the calculated actual power extracted from a GDL cavity. More details on this example can be found in Anderson (1972b).

Consider a gasdynamic laser cavity 58.5 cm wide in the beam direction (transverse to the flow) and 1.5 cm high. This size is representative of the NOL 3-megawatt arc tunnel after it was converted for gasdynamic laser experiments, as described by Anderson and Winkler (1971) and Anderson *et al.* (1971b). Consider also a very hypothetical Master Oscillator Power Amplifier (MOPA) arrangement (see Chapter X) consisting of a 1.5 $\times$ 10 cm rectangular beam transversing the cavity with five side-by-side passes beginning at the nozzle exit. Hence power is extracted over a cavity length of 50 cm. Assume that the input laser beam has a power P_{in} = 10kW with a Gaussian intensity distribution in the flow direction. Let P_{out} be the output power after the last pass. The power extracted from the gas is $P_e = P_{out} - P_{in}$. With this arrangement, the coupled power extraction, nonequilibrium gasdynamic analysis of Heiche and Harris (unpublished) yields the results shown in Table 4.1 for P_e.

For these results, the reservoir temperature and pressure were 1800°K and 37.5 atm, respectively, the mole fraction of CO_2 was 0.07, the nozzle area ratio was $A_e/A^* = 50$, and the nozzle throat height was $h^* = 0.3$ mm. Three cases with different H_2O mole fractions are shown in Table 4.1. These results show that, for a gasdynamic laser the size of the NOL 3-megawatt arc tunnel, P_c is on the order of $\frac{1}{2}$ the maximum available power at the nozzle exit. This serves to illustrate the difference between e_{max} and the actual power extracted.

Several approximate methods [see, for example Hoffman and Vlases (1972) and Rigrod (1965)] are available for predicting power output; these

TABLE 4.1

Comparison of Power Extraction with Maximum Power Available

X_{H_2O}	e_{max} (kJ/lb$_m$) at nozzle exit	$P_e/\dot{m}$ (kJ/lb$_m$)	Percent of maximum available
0.01	23.4	12.2	52
0.035	19.8	10.5	53
0.07	15.7	6.67	43

$\dot{m}$ = 1.5 lb/sec

are generally based on the estimation of saturation intensity within the cavity. However, for accurate results necessary for reasonable comparison between theory and experiment and for detailed gasdynamic laser design, a coupled numerical solution such as described above is required. Lee (1974) has very recently published details of a coupled power extraction analysis that uses the time-dependent approach described earlier. Because Lee's analysis is a natural continuation of our previous discussion, and because it is the first published fully coupled power extraction analysis, we will outline his approach. (Unpublished, coupled power extraction analyses have also been carried out by members of the Avco Everett Research Laboratory and the United Aircraft Research Laboratory, in addition to the Naval Ordnance Laboratory as mentioned earlier.)

Consider our previous discussion of the quasi-one-dimensional, time-dependent solution of gasdynamic laser flows. To extend the analysis for the case of power extraction, Lee has added a radiation term to the energy equation. Hence, Eq. (4.5) becomes

$$\frac{\partial e}{\partial t} = -\frac{p}{\rho}\left(\frac{\partial u}{\partial x} + u\,\frac{\partial \ln A}{\partial x}\right) - u\,\frac{\partial e}{\partial x} - Q_R \tag{4.21}$$

where Q_R is the laser energy emitted per unit mass of gas mixture. From the radiative transfer equation, Eq. (4.20),

$$dI_\nu/ds = G_\nu I_\nu \tag{4.22}$$

where s is measured in the direction of the radiative intensity. Equation (4.22) has dimensions of energy per second per unit volume; it physically represents the laser energy emitted per second per unit volume of gas.

Thus Q_R in Eq. (4.21) becomes

$$Q_R = G_\nu I_\nu/\rho \tag{4.23}$$

where G_ν is the local gain of the laser gas. Recall that G_ν is proportional to the local population inversion existing in the presence of the radiative intensity; hence it is distinctly different from the small-signal gain G_0, which assumes that the radiation field is so small that the kinetically generated population inversions are not affected by radiation. Thus $G_\nu < G_0$.

The continuity and momentum equations, Eqs. (4.3) and (4.4), remain unchanged. However, the rate equations must account for the laser radiative transitions from the (001) to the (100) levels in CO_2. The kinetic model shown in Fig. 3.4 must be employed. The model of Fig. 4.2 is no longer valid, since strong radiative emission pulls the (001) level out of local equilibrium with N_2. Referring to Fig. 3.2, laser emission *decreases* the population of the upper laser level (001) and *increases* the population of the lower level (100). Hence, referring to Eqs. (3.44)–(3.46), E_3 is decreased and E_{12} is increased by laser transitions. Since Eq. (4.23) gives the laser energy emitted per unit mass of *mixture*, then $G_\nu I_\nu/\rho_{CO_2}$ is the energy emitted per unit mass of CO_2, where ρ_{CO_2} is the local density of CO_2. Since ν_L is the frequency of the laser radiation, then $G_\nu I_\nu/h\nu_L\rho_{CO_2}$ is the number of radiative transitions per second per unit mass of CO_2, i.e., the number of molecules leaving the (001) level and arriving in the (100) level due strictly to the radiative transitions. Each molecule that leaves (001) reduces E_3 by $h\nu_3$; each molecule that arrives in (100) increases E_{12} by $h\nu_1$. Hence, for the case that includes laser radiation, Eq. (3.45) becomes

$$\begin{aligned}
\frac{dE_{12}}{dt} = {} & \frac{\nu_1 G_\nu I_\nu}{\nu_L \rho_{CO_2}} + 2\left[Z_{CC}P\overset{10}{(C2, C)} + Z_{CH}P\overset{10}{(C2, H)} + Z_{CN}P\overset{10}{(C2, N)}\right] \\
& \times \left[\exp(-\theta_2/T)\theta_2 R_{CO_2} - E_2(1 - \exp(-\theta_2/T))\right] \\
& + 3\theta_2 R_{CO_2}\left[Z_{CC}Q_C\overset{03}{\underset{10}{(C2, C3)}} + Z_{CH}Q_H\overset{03}{\underset{10}{(C2, C3)}} + Z_{CN}Q_N\overset{03}{\underset{10}{(C2, C3)}}\right] \\
& \times \left[\left(\frac{E_2}{\theta_2 R_{CO_2}} + 1\right)^3 \left(\frac{E_3}{\theta_3 R_{CO_2}}\right) - \exp[(3\theta_2 - \theta_3)/T]\right. \\
& \left. \times \left(\frac{E_3}{\theta_3 R_{CO_2}} + 1\right)\left(\frac{E_2}{\theta_2 R_{CO_2}}\right)^3\right]
\end{aligned} \tag{4.24}$$

and Eq. (3.46) becomes

$$\begin{aligned}\frac{dE_3}{dt} = {}& -\frac{\nu_3 G_\nu I_\nu}{\nu_L \rho_{\mathrm{CO_2}}} + \Big[Z_{\mathrm{CC}}Q_{\mathrm{C}} \overset{03}{\underset{10}{(\mathrm{C2, C3})}} + Z_{\mathrm{CH}}Q_{\mathrm{H}} \overset{03}{\underset{10}{(\mathrm{C2, C3})}} \\ & + Z_{\mathrm{CN}}Q_{\mathrm{N}} \overset{03}{\underset{10}{(\mathrm{C2, C3})}}\Big] \left[\exp[(3\theta_2-\theta_3)/T]\left(\frac{E_2}{\theta_2 R_{\mathrm{CO_2}}}\right)^3 (E_3+\theta_3 R_{\mathrm{CO_2}}) \right. \\ & \left. - E_3\left(\frac{E_3}{\theta_2 R_{\mathrm{CO_2}}}+1\right)^3\right] + Z_{\mathrm{CN}} Q \overset{01}{\underset{10}{(\mathrm{N, C3})}} \left[\exp(-(\theta_4-\theta_3)/T) \right. \\ & \left. \times \left(\frac{E_4}{\theta_4 R_{\mathrm{N_2}}}\right)(E_3+\theta_3 R_{\mathrm{CO_2}}) - E_3\left(\frac{E_4}{\theta_4 R_{\mathrm{N_2}}}+1\right)\right]\end{aligned} \tag{4.25}$$

Equation (3.44) for dE_4/dt remains unchanged. Therefore, for a quasi-one-dimensional, time-dependent, coupled power extraction analysis, Eqs. (3.44), (4.3), (4.4), (4.21), (4.23), (4.24), and (4.25) must be solved simultaneously. [As indicated by Anderson (1970a), the energy equation in terms of T rather than internal energy e is usually more convenient for nonequilibrium flow analyses because the transition probabilities and relaxation times depend explicitly on T. Equation (4.21) can be readily expressed in terms of T by using the fact that $e = e_{\mathrm{trans}} + e_{\mathrm{rot}} + e_{\mathrm{vib}} = \frac{5}{2}RT + e_{\mathrm{vib}}$.]

The time-dependent technique is the same as before; initial values for the radiative intensity I_ν, ρ, u, and T are assumed at $t = 0$, and the proper steady-state solution is obtained at large values of time. However, some boundary conditions or stipulations on I_ν must be imposed; this is where the actual cavity design comes into the analysis. Lee (1974) treated the case of a stable oscillator and imposed the condition that gain through the gas equals the loss at the mirrors on the boundary (the side-walls of the laser cavity). Lee notes that experimental measurements show that I_ν is relatively constant in the flow direction for stable resonators, and this allows the boundary condition to be applied as the average gain equals the average loss

$$\int_0^M (\ln r_1 r_2 - 2Gl)\, dx = 0 \tag{4.26}$$

where M is the mirror length, r_1 and r_2 are the mirror reflectivities, and l is the mirror separation distance. More information on cavity properties and design is given in Chapter X. It is sufficient to note here that Eq. (4.26) must be satisfied during the solution of the gasdynamic and kinetic rate equations and it serves to define uniquely the problem for a stable oscillator. Also note that I_ν does not appear explicitly in Eq. (4.26); rather, I_ν is implicit in G. I_ν affects the population inversions as reflected in Eqs. (4.24) and (4.25), hence G depends on I_ν. The value of I_ν is iterated until the resulting G (which varies with x) satisfies Eq. (4.26).

The properties of the laser gas flowing through the cavity are obviously affected by power extraction. Results calculated by Lee (1974) are shown in Figs. 4.13 and 4.14. Power extraction depletes the upper laser level, resulting in a rapid drop of T_4 and T_3 with distance through the cavity, as shown in Fig. 4.13. Correspondingly, the lower laser level is populated during power extraction, hence T_{12} increases with distance. Power is extracted most rapidly from the upstream portions of the cavity and less rapidly downstream, being limited by the pumping rate from N_2 to $CO_2(001)$. Thus, at the downstream locations, T_{12} once again tries to equilibrate with the translational temperature T. The translational temperature itself is increased during power extraction. This may sound strange at first thought; the gas is *loosing* energy due to laser emission, yet its temperature is *increasing*. However, recall that the source of laser radiation is the *nonequilibrium vibrational* energy of N_2 and CO_2 (ν_3) and that each CO_2 molecule, after giving up a photon of radiation, ultimately looses 1338 cm^{-1} of energy to the translational-rotational motion of the gas via the T–V deactivation of the combined ν_1 and ν_2 modes (see Figs. 3.2, 3.4, and 4.2). The temperature T is a reflection of the translational-rotational energy of the gas; as this energy is increased during power extraction, so is T. Referring to Fig. 4.14, laser power extraction causes a sharp decrease in

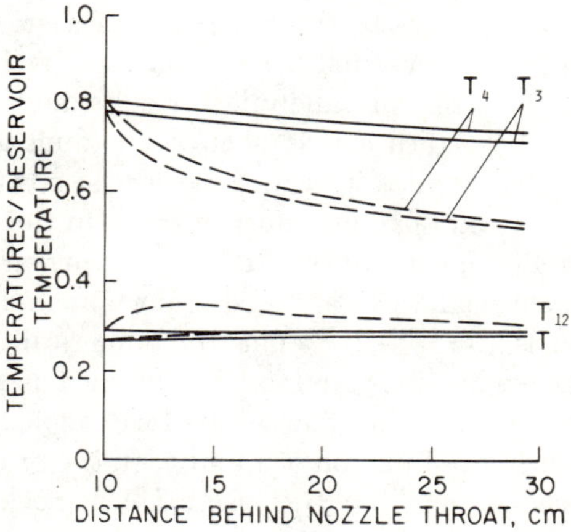

FIG. 4.13 Vibrational and static temperatures in the cavity with (---) and without (—) lasing. (After Lee, 1974.)

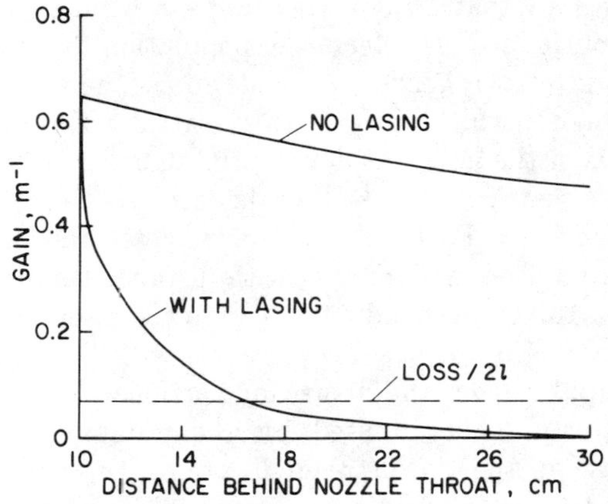

FIG. 4.14 Gain distributions in the cavity with and without lasing. (After Lee, 1974.)

the gain. The curve labeled "no lasing" corresponds to small-signal gain; the curve labeled "with lasing" is the actual loaded gain of the lasing gas as a function of distance along the cavity. The "gain equals loss" condition embodied in Eq. (4.26) is also illustrated in Fig. 4.14, where the areas under the gain and loss curves are equal.

Remember that Lee's analysis described above is one-dimensional. As the laser beam travels across the cavity, transverse to the flow, its intensity increases according to $dI_\nu = G_\nu I_\nu \, dy$, where y is the coordinate along the beam, perpendicular to x. Hence the laser beam will induce variations in the flow properties *transverse* to the flow; these variations are not taken into account by a one-dimensional analysis such as by Lee (1974). However, comparisons between his analytical results and experiment (discussed in Chapter V) indicate that such a one-dimensional analysis is sufficient for a stable resonator, where power is extracted through an array of small holes in an opaque copper mirror. On the other hand, for a Master Oscillator Power Amplifier (MOPA) arrangement (see Chapter X), such two-dimensional variations are important and should be taken into account. That is, $dI_\nu = G_\nu I_\nu \, dy$ must be numerically integrated point by point across the cavity, the gain must be obtained as a function of both x and y, and the corresponding flow properties coupled to the radiation must also be obtained as a function of x and y. In the process the variation of I_ν across the laser beam, $I_\nu = f(x)$, is obtained. Such detailed calculations have been made at the Naval Ordnance Laboratory, but the analysis and its results are not available in the literature. It is sufficient to state that two-dimensional effects are important for MOPA calculations.

In summary, this chapter has described techniques for calculating gasdynamic laser small-signal gain, maximum available energy, and coupled power extraction. How accurate are these techniques? How well can we really predict gasdynamic laser performance? The answers to these questions are the subject of the next chapter.

Chapter V

Comparison between Theory and Experiment

The previous chapters have provided the groundwork for an understanding of gasdynamic lasers. The basic physical principles have been discussed, and methods for the *calculation* of performance have been detailed. The results of such calculations given in Chapter IV clearly show that population inversions, laser gain, and laser power extraction can occur in supersonic expansions of CO_2–N_2–H_2O or He mixtures. These calculations have been generally confirmed by experiment, and such experiments are the subject of this chapter. The results shown in this chapter also draw heavily on the work of Anderson *et al.* (1971a, b) at the Naval Ordnance Laboratory (NOL).

5.1 Kinetic Rate Data

The vibrational relaxation times used to obtain the theory curves in this section are correlations of the data compiled in Taylor and Bitterman (1967), with the exception of the water rate $(\tau_c)_{CO_2-H_2O}$. Based on recent calculation by Sharman (1971), the present model assumes that $(\tau_c p)_{CO_2-H_2O}$ is constant for $T \leq 600°K$. This approximation is not good for $T < 200°K$, but such low temperatures are usually not encountered in the flows of interest here.

5.2 Nonequilibrium Gasdynamics

In the analysis of Anderson (1970c), the kinetic rate equations are fully coupled with the governing flow equations of continuity, momentum, and energy. Nonequilibrium conditions are included both upstream and downstream of the nozzle throat. The governing equations, along with their time-dependent numerical solution, have been described in Chapter IV. Hence no further elaboration will be given here.

5.3 Small-Signal Gain

The fundamental experimental measurement discussed in this section is the small-signal gain coefficient G_0, defined as $dI_\nu/I_\nu = G_0\, dx$. Here I_ν is the intensity of a low power CO_2 diagnostic laser beam at 10.6 μm incident on an element of gas of thickness (dx) in the supersonic flow, as shown schematically in Fig. 5.1. In principle, the intensity increase dI_ν yields a measurement of G_0. The intensity I_ν must be small enough such that the radiation field does not disturb the population inversion, i.e., such that (N_{001}–N_{100}) is collision dominated. In this case G_0 is directly proportional to the population inversion. A detailed discussion and derivation of the small-signal gain equation is given in Chapter II. With the appropriate rotational constants, a close approximation of Eq. (2.20) for the P(20) transition of the 10.6 band is

$$G_0 = \frac{\lambda^2}{4\pi\tau_{21}\nu_c}(N_{001}\text{–}N_{100})\left(\frac{45.6}{T}\right)e^{-234/T} \qquad (5.1)$$

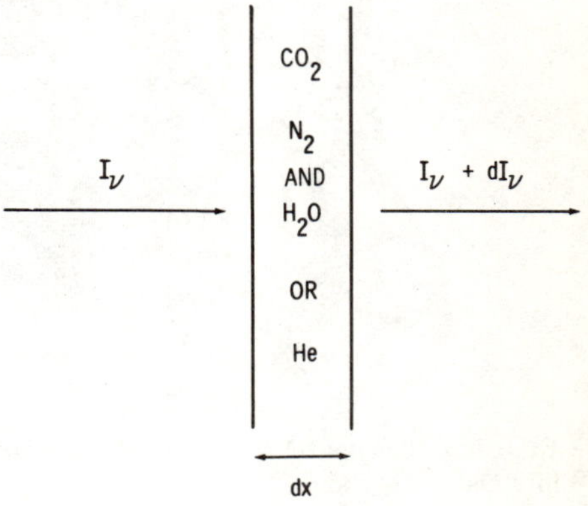

FIG. 5.1 Definition of small-signal gain coefficient. $dI_\nu/I_\nu = G_0\, dx$; $G_0 \propto (N_{001}\text{–}N_{100})$.

where $\lambda = 10.6 \times 10^{-6}$ m, τ_{21} is the spontaneous radiative lifetime equal to 5.38 sec, ν_c is the collision frequency, and T is in °K. Equation (5.1) assumes pressure line broadening only; Doppler broadening is negligible for the pressures of interest at the nozzle exit (50 Torr). The quantities in Eq. (5.1) are not limited to a specific set of units; however, they must be consistent, such as the SI system. The numerical constants in the last two factors have units of °K.

Thus theoretical vibrational population inversions (N_{001}–N_{100}) are obtained from the analysis of Chapter IV. In turn these are used in Eq. (5.1) to give theoretical predictions of G_0 for the P(20) transition of the 10.6 μm band. For other $P(J)$ transitions in the same band, Eq. (5.1) must be appropriately ratioed, assuming rotational equilibrium. The purpose of the remainder of this chapter is to compare the theoretically predicted G_0 with experimental measurements.

5.4 NOL 3-MW Arc Tunnel

The NOL 3-MW arc tunnel is an arc-heated, high-temperature, supersonic wind tunnel facility (Anderson and Winkler, 1971). The artist's conception in Fig. 5.2 shows the major conventional components of the wind tunnel. Electrical power is delivered from an ac power supply to the 4-ring 3-phase ac arc heater. Nitrogen (or air) is heated to the desired pres-

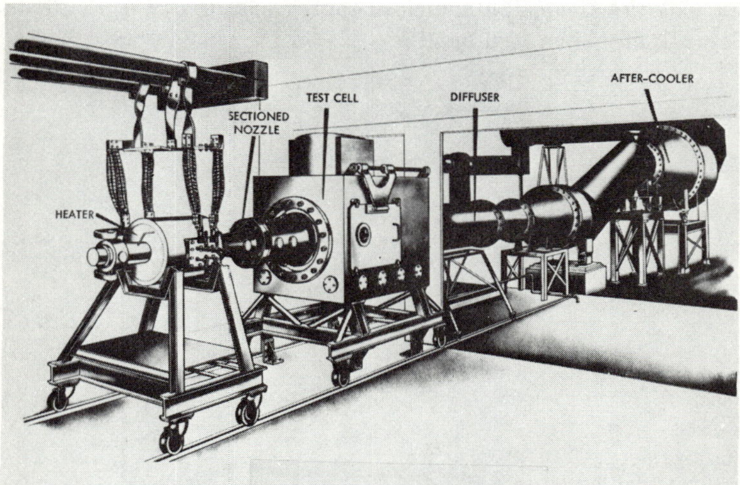

FIG. 5.2 Schematic of the 3-MW arc tunnel at the Naval Ordnance Laboratory, White Oak, Maryland.

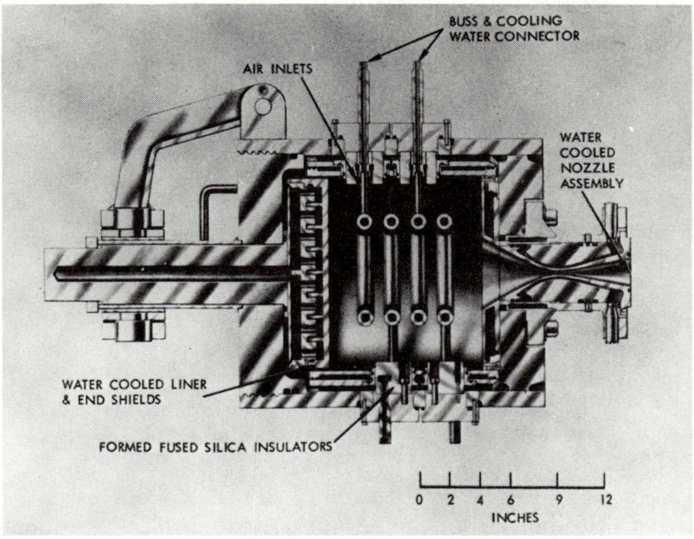

FIG. 5.3 Cross section of the MK IV arc heater at the Naval Ordnance Laboratory.

sure and temperature by the arc. In its conventional wind tunnel configuration, the high temperature gas passes through the supersonic nozzle into the test cell, where aerodynamic and heat transfer data are usually obtained. The gas then passes through the diffuser, an after-cooler, and to a vacuum pumping plant.

The arc heater (Winkler *et al.*, 1970) is of the 4-ring 3-phase ac type developed at the Naval Ordnance Laboratory (see Fig. 5.3). Water-cooled copper electrodes and liners are placed within the steel pressure shell. The gas to be heated is injected into the chamber through a series of holes around one leg of each electrode. The gas is heated by the two arc columns that (due to their self-induced magnetic field) rotate around the electrodes. The arc heater is capable of operation over a range of temperatures from 1500 to 6000°K and pressure of 10 to 70 atm. Extensive operating experience at pressures of 10 to 35 atm gives heater efficiencies of 25 to 60% depending upon the temperature and mass flow required.

For the small-signal gain measurements, the conventional arrangement shown in Fig. 5.2 is modified. Specifically, a mixing chamber, supersonic rapid expansion nozzle, and constant area duct are substituted for the conventional wind tunnel nozzle. This modified arrangement is shown in the schematic of Fig. 5.4 and the photo of Fig. 5.5. In the mixing chamber, CO_2 and liquid H_2O are injected and mixed with the hot N_2 from the arc heater. The hot gas mixture passes through the supersonic rapid expansion

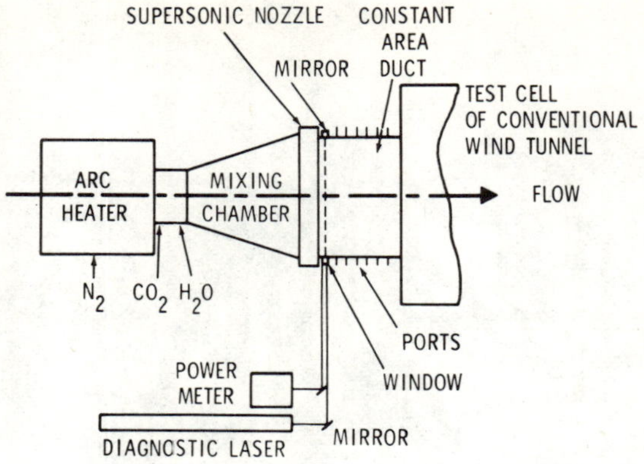

FIG. 5.4 Top view schematic of the NOL 3-MW arc tunnel modified as a gasdynamic laser.

nozzle, where the population inversion is created. The two-dimensional, contoured, minimum length nozzle has a throat height of 1 mm, an inviscid-core area ratio of 20, and a length transverse to the flow of 585 mm. The flow passes through an essentially constant area duct that is provided with a series of seven viewing ports along its length. The duct is slightly divergent to account for viscous effects. The output beam [10.6 μm,

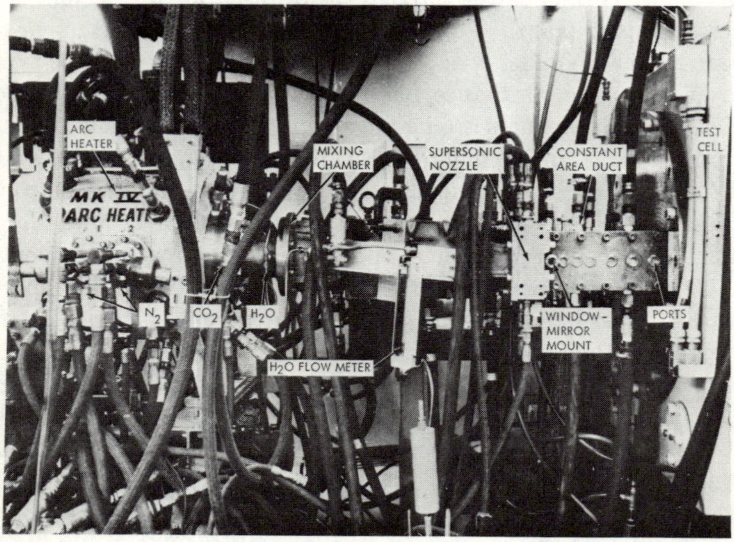

FIG. 5.5 The NOL 3-MW arc tunnel configured for small-signal gain measurements.

P(20) transition] from a homemade diagnostic CO_2 gas laser (see Fig. 5.6) is directed into the duct through an IRTRAN window, reflected from a gold-coated mirror on the opposite side of the duct, and passed back out the window into a broadband cw laser power meter (Coherent Radiation Labs Model 201). The small-signal gain along the duct may be measured by moving the window and mirrors so that the diagnostic laser beam passes through the desired point location.

The reservoir temperature of the gas mixture entering the supersonic nozzle is determined by use of a one-dimensional mass flow relationship from a sonic throat condition. The measured arc heater pressure and mass flows of the individual gases (N_2, CO_2, and H_2O) are used with specific heat ratios, compressibility factors, and gas constants for the mixture to calculate the nozzle reservoir temperature. The procedure is similar to that normally used in high-temperature wind tunnel systems (Warren, 1959).

The spectral output of the diagnostic CO_2 gas laser was measured with the aid of a Jarrell–Ash model (82000) spectrometer and a liquid nitrogen-cooled detector. The laser was found to operate predominantely on the P(20) transition; the P(18) and P(16) transitions also occurred but were weak enough to be ignored in the small-signal gain measurements and in the analytical calculations.

The sequence of events leading to a small-signal gain measurement is as

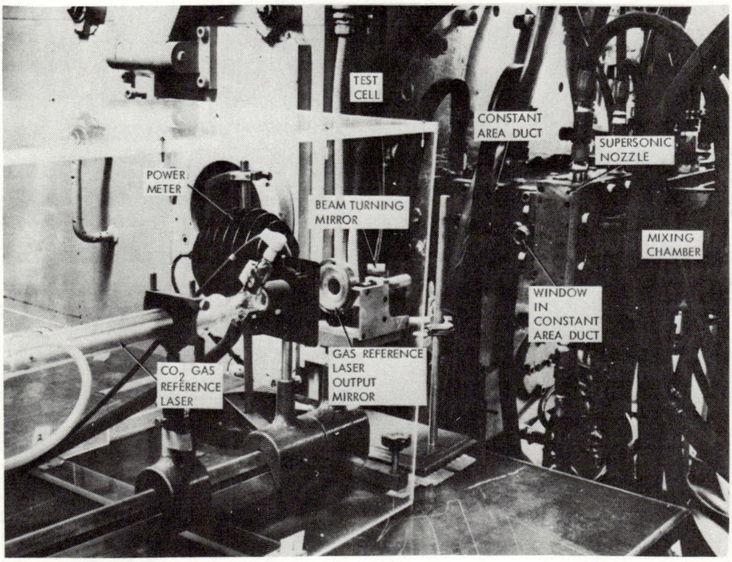

FIG. 5.6 The optical arrangement for measuring small-signal gain.

follows. First, the diagnostic laser and optical system are aligned to give the maximum power incident on the power meter. Then, the arc heater is turned on, heating pure N_2 at a temperature somewhat above the final reservoir temperature. When steady flow conditions are reached in the heater, cold CO_2 and liquid H_2O are injected into the mixing chamber (see Figs. 5.4 and 5.5). The power meter continuously records the power level of the beam after it has doubly traversed the duct. The beam power W_1 measured during the steady flow of the N_2–CO_2–H_2O mixture and the power W_0 measured during the preliminary flow of pure N_2 yield G_0 from the relationship $W_1/W_0 = \exp(G_0L)$, where L is the geometric path length inside the duct.

5.5 NOL 12.7-cm Shock Tunnel

The arc tunnel discussed above is one means of providing a reservoir of hot, vibrationally excited gas for subsequent expansion through a nozzle. Another means is to utilize the shock-heated gas behind a reflected shock wave in a shock tube. In the present experiments, a conventional pressure-driven shock tube is used to provide reservoir conditions behind a reflected shock wave in a mixture of CO_2–N_2–He. A nonequilibrium population inversion is created when this shock-heated mixture expands through a nozzle mounted at the end of the tube. The flow then passes through a slightly diverging cavity, where measurements of G_0 are made, and finally

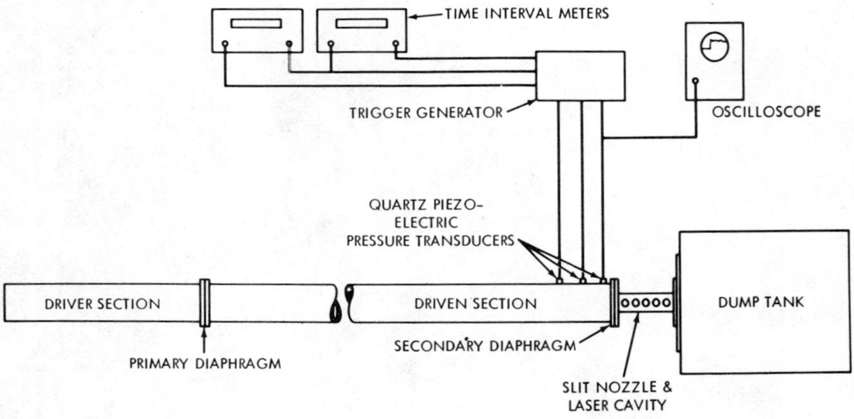

FIG. 5.7 Schematic of the 12.7-cm shock tunnel gasdynamic laser facility at the Naval Ordnance Laboratory.

exhausts into an evacuated dump tank. Some features of the experimental apparatus are given below, and a schematic of the shock tube arrangement is given in Fig. 5.7.

The shock tube is 12.7 cm in diameter and utilizes a single diaphragm to separate the driver and driven sections. The driven section terminates with an end wall plate and a 0.077-mm-thick brass diaphragm to separate the nozzle from the driven section prior to the performance of an experiment. During operation of the shock tube, the incident shock wave reflects from the end plate, produces stagnation conditions for operation of the nozzle, and ruptures the secondary diaphragm. Uniform flow is maintained through the nozzle for about 1 msec. The nozzle is a minimum length, two-dimensional, contoured slit nozzle with a 1 mm throat height and an inviscid core area ratio of 20. The nozzle width is 12.7 cm. A detailed drawing of the shock tube end wall, nozzle, and cavity is shown in Fig. 5.8.

The shock tube was driven with cold helium in these experiments. A 5.88% CO_2–55% N_2–39.12% He mixture commercially obtained from the Matheson Company is used as the test gas. This gas mixture is supplied with an accuracy of ±2% of each component. The total impurities, as stated by Matheson, are less than 200 ppm and the H_2 and H_2O content are

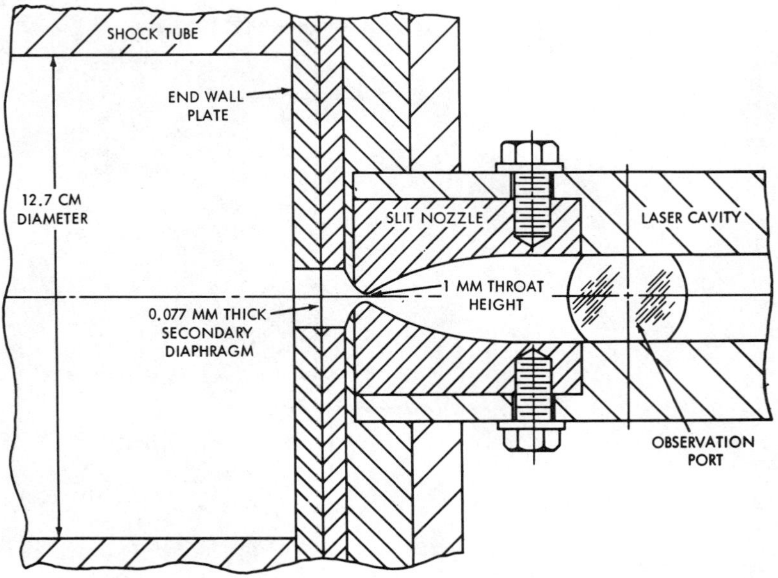

FIG. 5.8 Slit nozzle and laser cavity arrangement for the NOL 12.7-cm shock tunnel gasdynamic laser.

each stated as less than 50 ppm. Prior to filling the shock tube with the test gas mixture, it is evacuated to less than 10^{-3} Torr.

Experiments were performed for stagnation pressures of 19.47 to 23.56 atm and a range of stagnation temperatures from 1175 to 2240°K. The stagnation conditions are calculated from normal shock relationships assuming local thermodynamic equilibrium using the method of Madden *et al.* (1970) and the measured shock wave speed. Figure 5.7 shows the instrumentation for the measurement of the shock wave speed. Three quartz piezoelectric pressure transducers (manufactured by PCB Piezotronics, Inc.) and electronic counters are used to measure shock wave transit times. Pressure is measured using the transducer nearest the end wall.

Small-signal gain measurements are made downstream of the nozzle in the laser cavity. Five ports are spaced along the length of the cavity to enable longitudinal G_0 profiles to be made. G_0 is measured by directing the beam of a low-power diagnostic laser through the cavity and measuring the increase in power between no flow and flow conditions. A schematic of the instrumentation for measurements of small-signal gain is shown in Fig. 5.9.

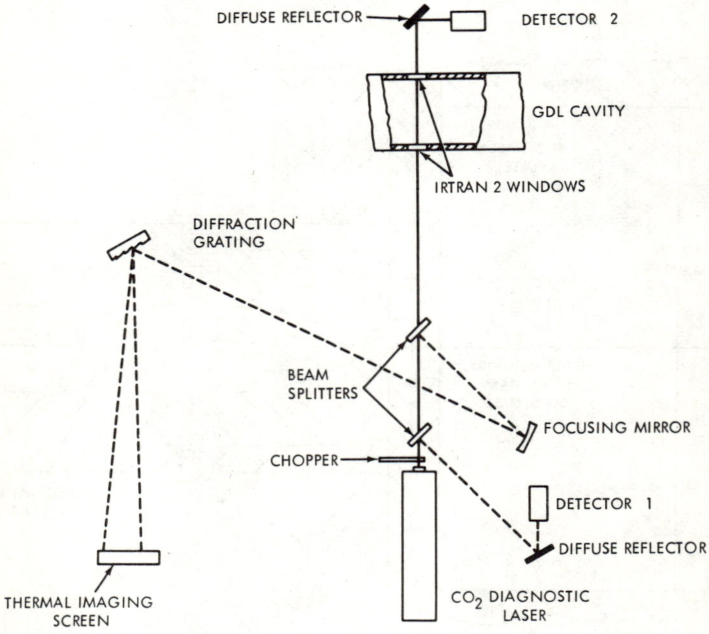

FIG. 5.9 Schematic of instrumentation for the measurement of small-signal gain in the NOL shock tunnel gasdynamic laser.

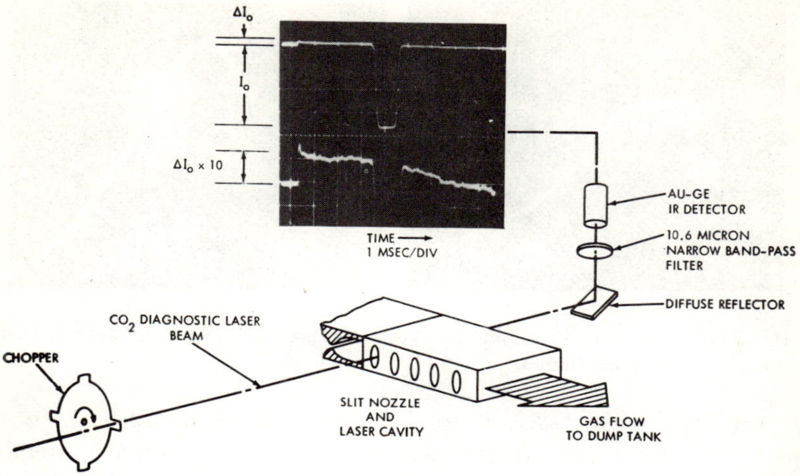

FIG. 5.10 Typical oscillograph trace from the shock tunnel gain measurements.

The diagnostic laser is a Sylvania Model 948 CO_2 laser. The beam is first mechanically chopped to establish a reference level and then sampled (by means of beam splitters) to determine wavelength and amplitude stability. One sampled beam is directed to a focusing mirror that reflects it to a grating blazed at 10 μm. This beam is dispersed by the grating and projected on to an OptEngineering thermal imaging screen, which displays the individual line or lines present and their corresponding mode structures. The second sampled beam is monitored by detector 1 to determine the amplitude stability of the diagnostic laser. The main probe beam passes through the windows (IRTRAN 2, antireflection coated) of the cavity and is then diffused by reflection from a rough surfaced aluminum flat to ensure coverage of the active area of the detector 2. A narrow-band-pass filter is inserted in the beam path to prevent extraneous radiation from invalidating the gain measurement. Detectors 1 and 2 are gold-doped germanium photoconductive cells operated at 77°K.

Figure 5.10 shows a typical oscilloscope trace of the probe beam as detected during an experiment. The lower trace is a 10× amplification of the upper trace. An upstream pressure transducer triggered the oscilloscope. The flat initial portion of the oscilloscope trace is representative of a no-flow condition in the cavity. The increase in signal indicates the start of flow in the cavity. (The upward deflection is indicative of gain.). The rectangular pulse is the chopped signal. The reference is indicated by I_0 and the increase in intensity by ΔI. The value of G_0 is given by

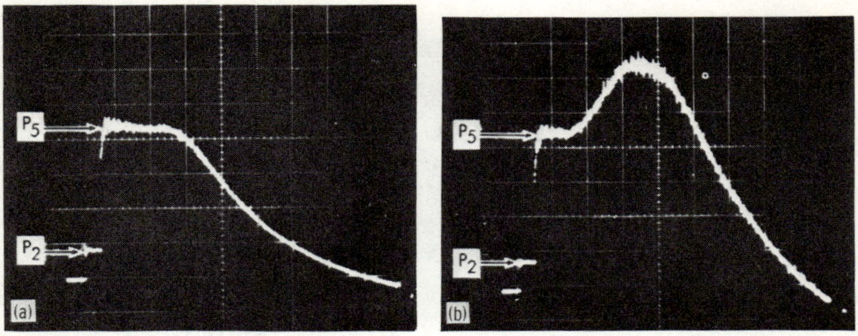

FIG. 5.11 Typical oscillograph traces of static pressure behind the reflected shock wave in the NOL shock tunnel.

$(I_0 + \Delta I)/I_0 = \exp(G_0 L)$, where L is the geometric path length (in this case, 12.7 cm for a single tranverse of the cavity). The gain measurements were made on the P(28) and P(30) lines. These lines [rather than the usual P(20) line] were used because the diagnostic laser was more stable at these transitions due to mirror misalignment within the laser.

Typical pressure records near the end wall are shown in Fig. 5.11. The initial abrupt pressure increase occurs when the incident shock wave passes over the pressure transducer. The second large pressure increase occurs as the reflected shock wave sweeps over the gauge. A pressure plateau persists for approximately 1 msec and is subsequently destroyed by wave interactions. Two types of wave interactions are shown in Fig. 5.11. Figure 5.11a is a pressure trace of conditions where the reflected head of the expansion wave, generated by the rupture of the primary diaphragm, eventually interacts with the reflected shock wave. The expansion wave lowers the pressure and cools the gas and thus terminates the test after about a millisecond running time. By comparison, Fig. 5.11b represents the interaction of the reflected shock wave with the contact surface and the subsequent generation of shock waves that are transmitted back into the stagnation region. These weaker shock waves cause the additional pressure and temperature increase in the nozzle reservoir region, which occurs after about 1 msec of useful test time. Eventually the pressure rapidly decays, which is indicative of the arrival of the expansion wave.

5.6 Arc Tunnel Experiments

Considering CO_2–N_2–H_2O mixtures, small-signal gain measurements have been obtained in the NOL 3-MW arc tunnel as a function of distance from the nozzle throat. A measured G_0 profile is shown in Fig. 5.12, where it is compared with the theoretically predicted profile obtained from the analysis of Anderson (1970c). Very good agreement is obtained. The slight drop of the experimental data below the theoretical curve at large downstream distances is to be expected. The real flow is influenced by boundary layer growth and weak oblique shock patterns in the constant area section, whereas the theoretical analysis assumes an inviscid, shock-free flow. The existance of a weak shock pattern has been experimentally observed (Greenberg *et al.*, 1970; Wagner, 1971.) In fact, a detailed experimental investigation of the fluid dynamics of short, minimum length nozzles is described by Wagner (1971).

Referring to Fig. 5.12, the initially rapid increase in G_0 as a function of distance is due to the rapid depopulation of the (100) CO_2 level by H_2O. The (001) level is also being depopulated, but at a slower rate. The peak gain is reached when N_{100} essentially equilibrates with T. Downstream of the peak, G_0 decreases due to the continuous deactivation of the (001) level. The different rates of relaxation for the (001) and (100) levels are clearly evident in Fig. 5.13, where theoretical results for the two vibrational temperatures and the translational temperature are shown as functions of distance along the duct.

In addition, the G_0 measured at a fixed station (1.9 cm downstream of the nozzle exit) is shown in Fig. 5.14 as a function of reservoir temperature. Again, the measurements are compared with theoretical predictions based on Anderson (1970c) and again reasonable agreement is obtained.

Examining Fig. 5.14, at lower temperatures G_0 increases rapidly with T_0 simply because the total vibrational energy in the reservoir increases. However, the relaxation rates also increase with temperature. Moreover, for a nozzle of fixed area ratio, the exit static temperature increases as T_0

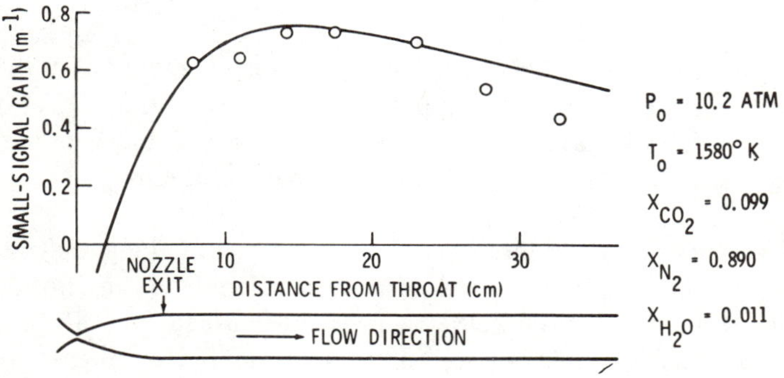

FIG. 5.12 Comparison between theoretical (—) and experimental (○) small-signal gain profiles.

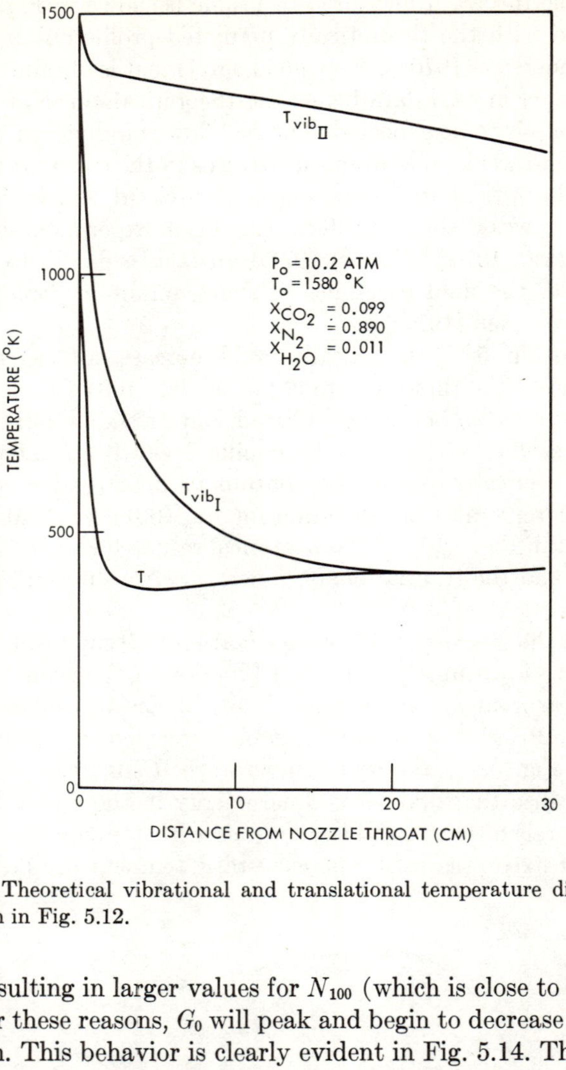

FIG. 5.13 Theoretical vibrational and translational temperature distributions for the case shown in Fig. 5.12.

increases, resulting in larger values for N_{100} (which is close to equilibration with T). For these reasons, G_0 will peak and begin to decrease if T_0 is made large enough. This behavior is clearly evident in Fig. 5.14. The magnitude and location of the peak depends on nozzle shape and size, p_0, and mixture ratio.

All of the previous measurements have been made along the centerline of the flow. The minimum length, two-dimensional nozzle employed for these measurements is contoured to provide uniform flow at the nozzle exit. Because the flow field is two-dimensional, the fluid elements traveling along different stream lines experience different flow gradients; thus the nonequilibrium history of each streamline is different. This prompts a

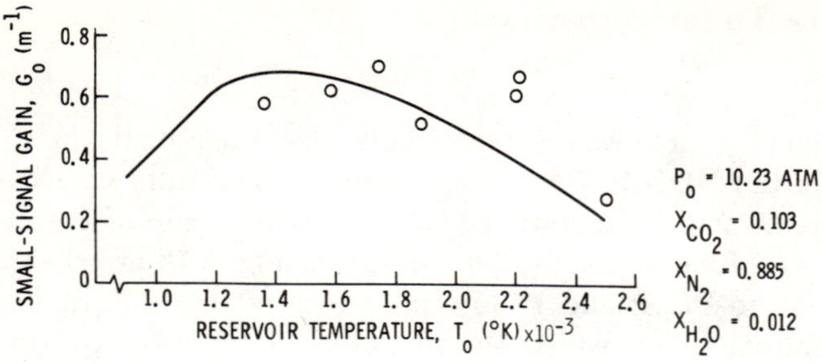

FIG. 5.14 Variation of small-signal gain with reservoir temperature; comparison between theory (—) and the NOL arc tunnel (○) data.

question regarding the uniformity of G_0 vertically across the nozzle exit. In order to investigate this question, measurements of G_0 were made off the centerline in a direction normal to the flow at a station 1.9 cm downstream of the nozzle exit. These measurements are shown in Fig. 5.15 and demonstrate a remarkably uniform G_0 distribution across the entire inviscid flow region. These off-centerline gain measurements are believed to be the first of their kind and indicate that two-dimensional effects are not serious for such internal nonequilibrium nozzle flows.

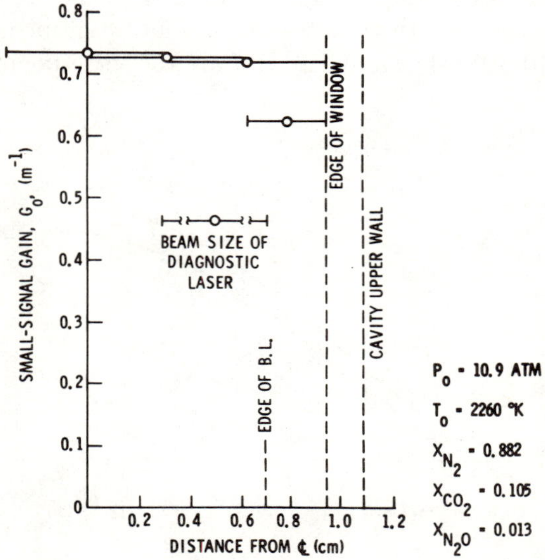

FIG. 5.15 Variation of small-signal gain transverse to the flow at a station 1.9 cm downstream of the nozzle exit in the NOL 3-MW arc tunnel.

5.7 . Shock Tunnel Experiments

Small-signal gain measurements have also been made in CO_2–N_2–He mixtures in the NOL 12.7-cm shock tunnel. The results are shown in Fig. 5.16, where G_0 at a fixed station (1.27 cm downstream of the nozzle exit) is plotted as a function of T_0. Also shown in Fig. 5.16 are theoretical predictions for the P(28) and P(30) transitions of the 10.6 μm band. These are the transitions on which the diagnostic laser was operating for the present shock tunnel experiments, as discussed earlier. Again, the theory based on Anderson (1970c) yields reasonable agreement with experiment, with the exception of the higher temperature range where the measured data fall slightly below theory. It is interesting to note that the equilibrium reservoir conditions for the present measurements indicate 1% dissociation for CO_2 at $T_0 = 2000°K$, growing to 5% at $T_0 = 2250°K$. The theoretical results shown in Fig. 5.16 assume a nonreacting, constant composition mixture and hence do not account for the partial dissociation of CO_2. This contributes in part to the over-prediction of G_0 at temperatures above 2000°K.

Small-signal gain measurements for CO_2–N_2–He mixtures have also been made in a shock tunnel by Christiansen and Tsongas (1971) at the University of Washington. Some of these data are shown in Fig. 5.17, where G_0 is plotted over a wide range of p_0. The measurements were made at the exit of a wedge nozzle with throat height 2 mm, total included angle 30°, and $A_e/A^* = 10$. Also shown in Fig. 5.17 are the corresponding theoretical

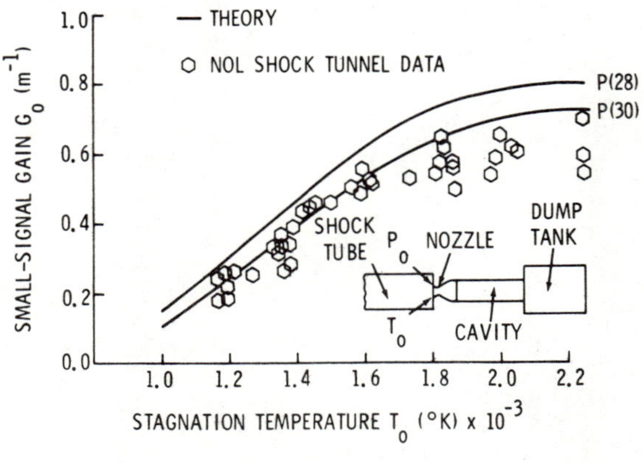

FIG. 5.16 Variation of small-signal gain with reservoir temperature. Comparison between theory (—) and experiment (○) at a station 1.27 cm downstream of the nozzle exit in the NOL shock tunnel: $p_0 = 20$ atm; $X_{CO_2} = 0.0588$, $X_{He} = 0.3912$, $X_{N_2} = 0.55$.

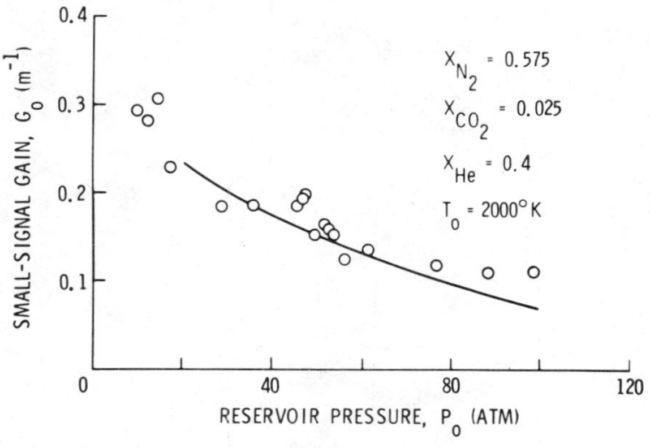

FIG. 5.17 Variation of small-signal gain with reservoir pressure. Comparison between theory (—; Anderson *et al.*, 1971a) and experiment (○; Christiansen and Tsongas, 1971).

predictions from the analysis of Anderson (1970c). Reasonable agreement is obtained between theory and experiment.

5.8 Other Experiments

A complete set of GDL arc tunnel experiments have been reported by Lee and Gowen (1971) and Lee *et al.* (1972). They give comparisons between theory and experiment for small-signal gain and laser power for CO_2–N_2–He and H_2O mixtures. The nozzle arrangement was an array of 24 Mach 4 nozzles of 1 mm throat height, in contrast to the single-slit nozzles described in the Naval Ordnance Laboratory experiments. Some of their results for small-signal gain are shown in Figs. 5.18–5.23, and some power data are shown in Figure 5.24. In these figures, the theoretical gain is obtained from the method of Anderson (1970c). Fairly reasonable agreement is obtained. The theoretical curves (the solid curves) for power in Figure 5.24 were obtained from an approximate analysis based on Rigrod (1965) for various values of mirror absorptivity. The actual mirror absorptivity in these experiments is not known, and Figure 5.24 illustrates the tenuous nature of power extraction analyses.

Another set of arc tunnel GDL experiments were performed by Howgate *et al.* (1972), who compared the experimental results with their detailed numerical calculations of laser power output. Discrepancies between theory and experiment ranged from 7 to 100%. This again illustrates the dif-

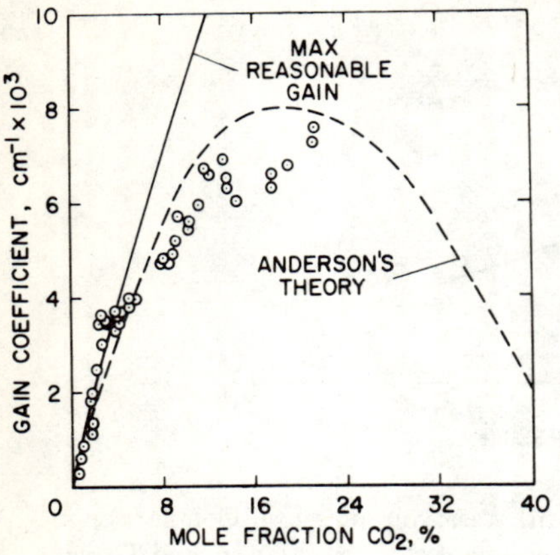

FIG. 5.18

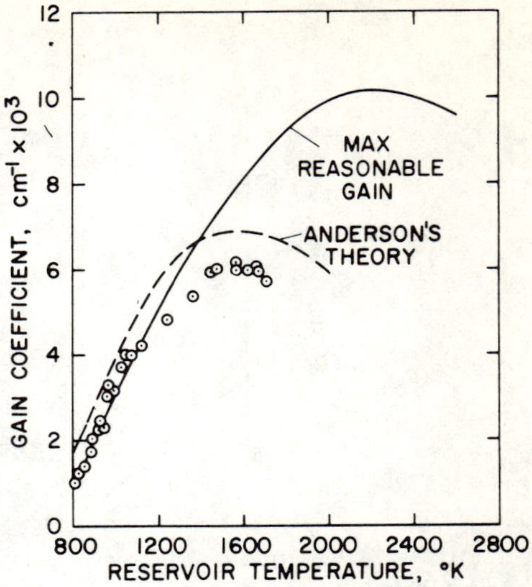

FIG. 5.19

FIG. 5.18 Effect of CO_2 concentration on small-signal gain. $He/N_2 = 0.65$; $T_0 = 1250°K$; $p_0 = 9$ atm. (After Lee *et al.*, 1972.)

FIG. 5.19 Effect of reservoir temperature on small-signal gain for a gas mixture of 6.5% CO_2, 39.5% He, and 54% N_2. $p_0 = 9$ atm. (After Lee *et al.*, 1972.)

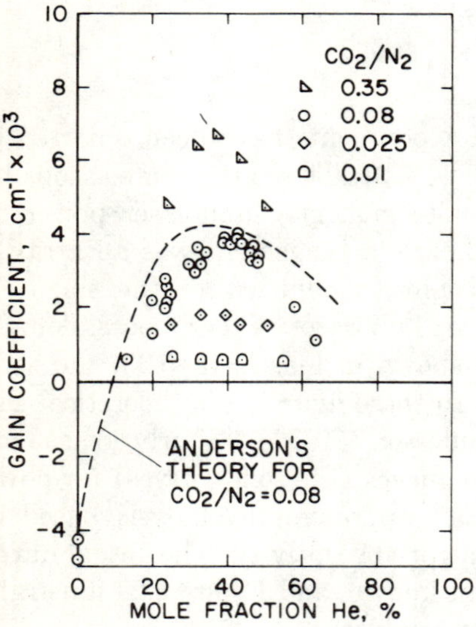

FIG. 5.20

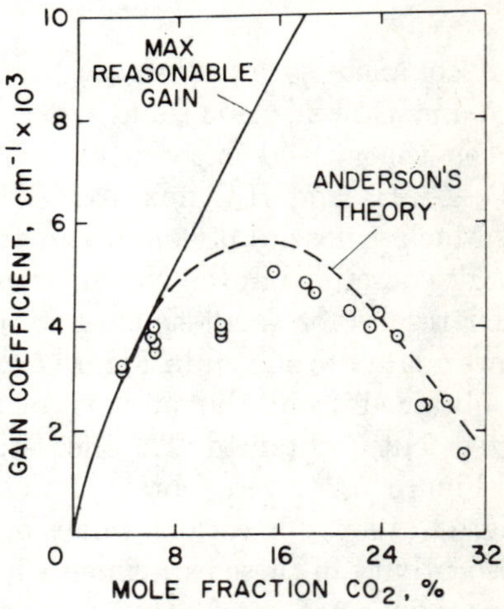

FIG. 5.21

FIG. 5.20 Effect of helium concentration on small-signal gain. $T_0 = 1250°K$; $p_0 = 9$ atm. (After Lee *et al.*, 1972.)

FIG. 5.21 Effect of CO_2 concentration on small-signal gain with 2.4% H_2O in the mixture. $T_0 = 1175°K$; $p_0 = 9$ atm. (After Lee *et al.*, 1972.)

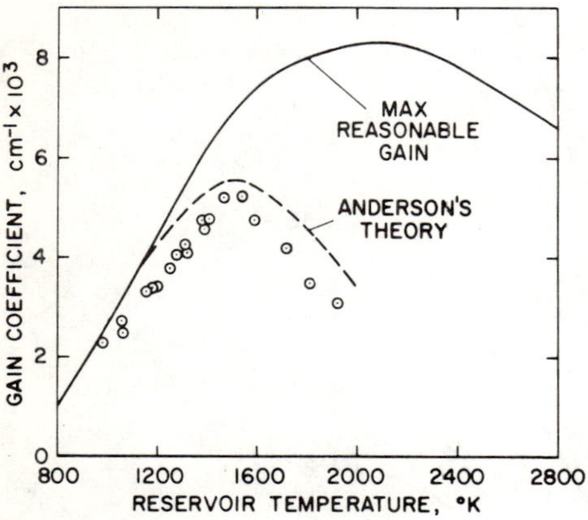

FIG. 5.22

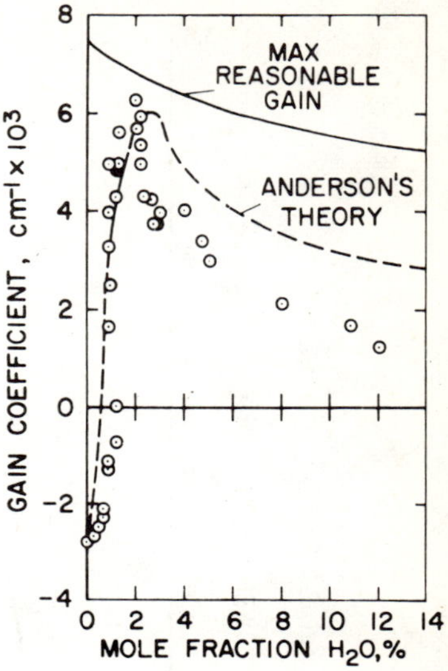

FIG. 5.23

FIG. 5.22 Effect of reservoir temperature on small-signal gain with a mixture of 2.4% H_2O, 6.3% CO_2, and 91.3% N_2. p_0 = 9 atm. (After Lee *et al.*, 1972.)

FIG. 5.23 Effect of H_2O concentration on small-signal gain with a constant 6.3% CO_2. T_0 = 1500°K; p_0 = 9 atm. (After Lee *et al.*, 1972.)

ficulties involved in accurately predicting power extraction in a GDL cavity.

Finally, with regard to conventional GDL arc tunnel experiments, McLeary (1972) reports "approximate" agreement between his theoretical calculations and the arc tunnel results presented by Anderson and Winkler (1971).

Other shock tunnel experiments are reported by Klosterman and Hoffman (1973), Christiansen and Tsongas (1971), Hertzberg *et al.* (1972), Vamos (1974), Tennant *et al.* (1974), Kuehn and Monson (1970), Biriukov *et al.* (1971), Sato and Sekiguchi (1973), and Gembarzhevskiy *et al.* (1972). Throughout all of these, comparison between theory and experiment ranges from poor to very good.

At this point the reader is reminded that a conventional gasdynamic laser operates with an equilibrium mixture of CO_2, N_2, and H_2O or He in the reservoir, independently of the way in which this hot, high-pressure mixture is obtained. It can be formed in an electric arc or by means of shock heating, as previously described, or it can also be formed by chemical

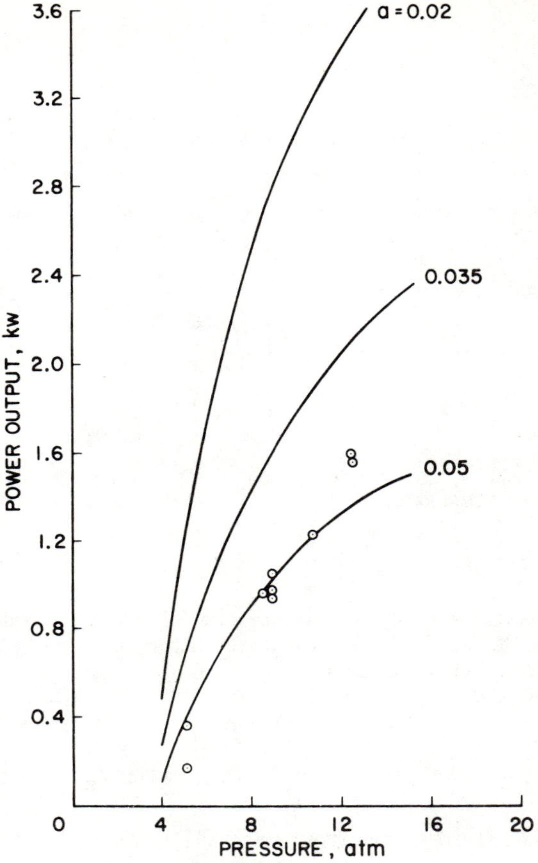

FIG. 5.24 Effect of reservoir pressure on power output. T_0 = 1350°K; 13% CO_2; 45% He; 42% N_2. (After Lee *et al.*, 1972.)

combustion, as initially reported by Gerry (1970). Several combustion-driven GDLs have been reported by Gerry (1970), Tulip and Sequin (1971), Yatsiv *et al.* (1971), Meinzer (1972), and Gabai *et al.* (1972). In each of these, comparisons are made with theory, and various degrees of agreement are again obtained. Of particular interest are the extensive parametric tests of Meinzer (1972), including the effect of H_2O on GDL gain all the way to 50% H_2O content. Meinzer compares his experimental data with results obtained from the analysis of Anderson (1970c), showing some reasonable agreement.

The most recent comparison between experimental measurements of

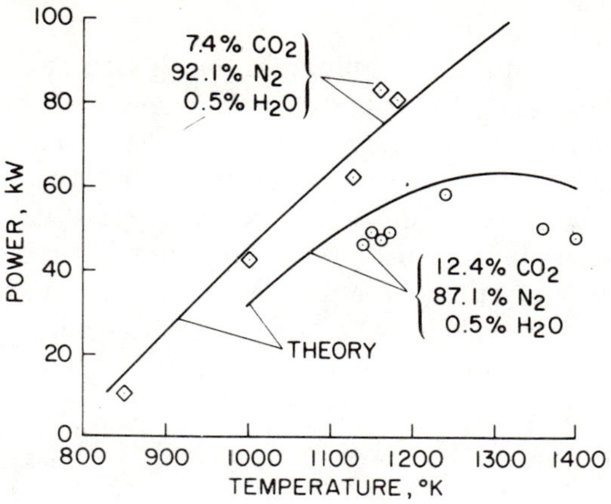

FIG. 5.25 Comparison of theory with experiment for power output from a combustion-driven gasdynamic laser. (After Lee, 1974.)

power extraction and theory is that of Lee (1974) for a combustion-driven gasdynamic laser with a stable resonator. This comparison is shown in Figs. 5.25 and 5.26, where the theory curves are obtained from the coupled power extraction analysis described at the end of Chapter IV. Here reasonable agreement between theory and experiment is obtained; this is a testi-

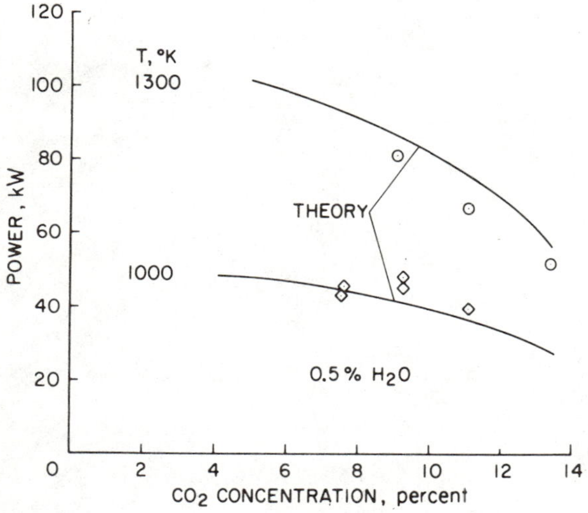

FIG. 5.26 Another comparison of theory and experiment for power output from a combustion-driven gasdynamic laser. (After Lee, 1974.)

monial to the necessity of coupling both the gasdynamics and the radiation in an analysis of power extraction.

A final remark is in order concerning the comparison of theory with experiment. Anderson (1973, 1974) has recently reported that, based on the current discrepancies in the existing rate data, a maximum uncertainty of 25 to 30% can be expected in any calculation of gasdynamic laser performance. These thoughts are given in detail in Appendix A. Also, in addition to uncertainties in the kinetic rates, any comparison between theory and experiment is subject to error due to shock wave and viscous flow effects in the laser cavity. Such effects are generally not included in the existing theoretical analyses.

Chapter VI

Inversions behind Normal Shock Waves

Basov and Oraevskii (1963) suggested that population inversions in molecular systems could be obtained by rapid *heating* of the system, as well as by rapid cooling as in the case of the conventional gasdynamic laser. One of the most rapid ways of heating a gas is by means of a shock wave. Therefore let us examine the purely vibrational relaxation process behind a normal shock wave in CO_2–N_2–He mixtures and assess what inversions, if any, occur in the nonequilibrium flow. This problem has been examined by Anderson and Madden (1971) and Anderson *et al.* (1970); the material for this chapter is drawn primarily from these references.

Consider the gasdynamic flow model shown in Fig. 6.1. We make the standard assumptions of a stationary, discontinuous shock front with frozen conditions immediately behind the front. Hence at this location ρ_2, T_2, and u_2 are obtained from the standard calorically perfect gas equations for normal shocks, and $e_{\mathrm{vib_I}}$ and $e_{\mathrm{vib_{II}}}$ are equal to their respective upstream values. In turn these quantities are the boundary conditions for the downstream nonequilibrium flow, which is solved by forward numerical integration of the governing steady flow conservation equations as functions of distance behind the shock front. These equations are:

Continuity

$$u \frac{d\rho}{dx} + \rho \frac{du}{dx} = 0 \qquad (6.1)$$

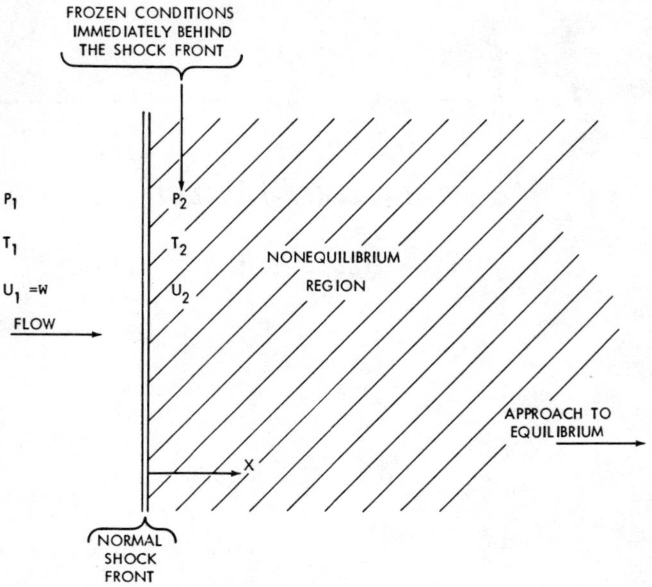

FIG. 6.1 Gasdynamic flow model for the nonequilibrium normal shock problem.

Momentum

$$(RT/\rho)\frac{d\rho}{dx} + R\,dT/dx + u\frac{du}{dx} = 0 \tag{6.2}$$

Energy

$$RT\frac{du}{dx} + uR\alpha\frac{dT}{dx} + u\frac{d}{dx}(e_{\text{vib}_\text{I}} + e_{\text{vib}_\text{II}}) = 0 \tag{6.3}$$

Rate

$$\frac{de_{\text{vib}_\text{I}}}{dx} = \frac{\dot{u}_\text{I}}{u} \quad \text{and} \quad \frac{de_{\text{vib}_\text{II}}}{dx} = \frac{\dot{u}_\text{II}}{u} \tag{6.4}$$

where $\alpha = \frac{3}{2}X_{\text{He}} + \frac{5}{2}(X_{\text{CO}_2} + X_{\text{N}_2})$, $p = \rho RT$, and the notation is standard. The solution is terminated when equilibrium values of the normal shock properties are closely approached. Equilibrium normal shock properties for CO_2–N_2–He mixtures are known in advance from Madden *et al.* (1970). A detailed discussion of the numerical aspects of the present study can be found in Anderson *et al.* (1970).

Numerical results for a typical case are shown in Figs. 6.2 and 6.3. Figure 6.2 illustrates temperature variations in the nonequilibrium region behind the shock front and clearly shows the rapid equilibration of $T_{\mathrm{vib_I}}$ with the translational temperature T, whereas in contrast $T_{\mathrm{vib_{II}}}$ relaxes more slowly. At a distance of 4 mm downstream of the shock front, all three temperatures have equilibrated within 1% of the final equilibrium temperature, which has been taken from the results of Madden *et al.* (1970). The results shown in Fig. 6.2 reflect a molecular collisional process that indeed leads to population inversions behind the shock front, as shown in Fig. 6.3. These inversions occur between the (040) and (001) levels and to a lesser degree between the (200) and (001) levels in CO_2. Examining Fig. 6.3, near the shock front the inversions rapidly increase owing to the rapid population of the excited levels of mode I while at the same time the excitation of mode II is lagging far behind. However, the inversion soon peaks and begins to decrease farther downstream as the lower (001) level is substantially populated. Note that, for the given upstream conditions, the inversions persist over a length from 1 to 2 mm behind the shock front. The vibrational kinetics obey binary scaling; hence the spatial extent of the population inversions can be increased or decreased by a proportional decrease or increase in p_1, keeping T_1 and u_1 the same. Many additional results obtained from the present study are discussed in Anderson *et al.* (1970).

How do the laser properties of this nonequilibrium shock flow compare

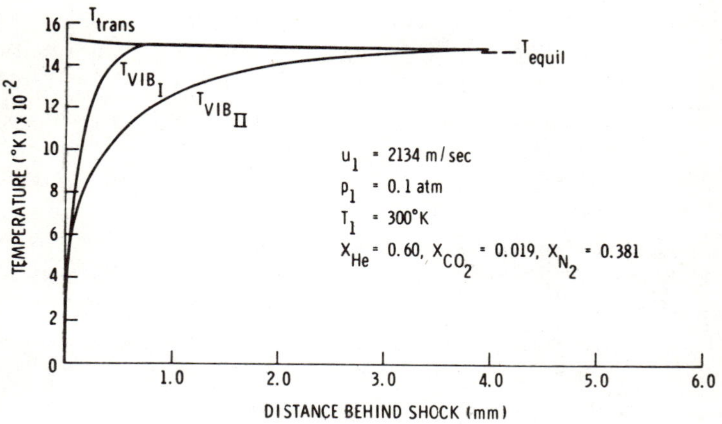

FIG. 6.2 Variation of translational and vibrational temperatures with distance behind a normal shock front in a CO_2–N_2–He mixture. (After Anderson and Madden, 1971.)

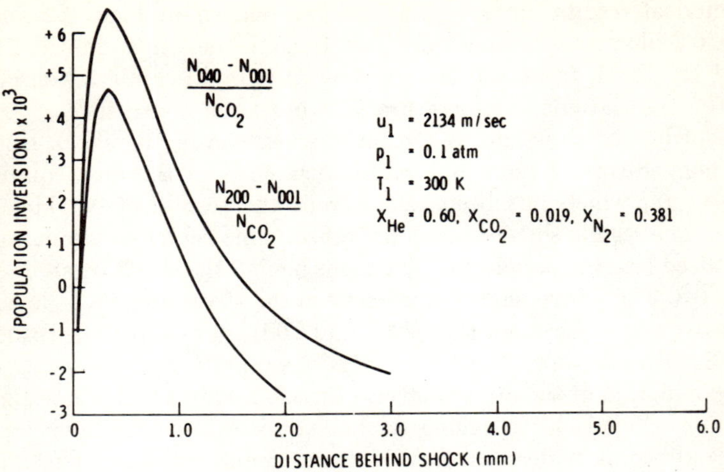

FIG. 6.3 Variation of population inversions behind the shock front.

with those obtained by rapid expansions? First, the conventional, rapid expansion gasdynamic laser creates a population inversion between the (001) and (100) levels in CO_2 that subsequently lases at $\lambda = 10.6\ \mu m$. In contrast, the inversions shown in Fig. 6.3 between the (040) and (001) levels and between the (200) and (001) levels would correspond to laser transitions at 50 μm and 22 μm, respectively. An important parameter for gas lasers is small-signal gain G_0 defined in Chapter II. From our previous discussion, $G_0 \propto (\lambda^2/\tau_{21})\ IN \propto (M^2/\lambda)\ IN$, where τ_{21} is the spontaneous radiative lifetime for a transition between the upper and lower laser levels, M is the corresponding quantum mechanical matrix element, and IN is the population inversion. For CO_2, computed values of M for the 50 μm, 22 μm, and 10.6 μm transitions are in the ratio 0.21×10^{-2}:0.21×10^{-2}:0.34×10^{-1}, respectively (from G. Lalos, unpublished, Naval Ordnance Laboratory). Also, the shock-induced population inversions shown in Fig. 6.3 are approximately one order of magnitude smaller than typical inversions created in rapid expansion through supersonic nozzles. In light of the above numbers, a comparison of G_0 at 50 μm and 22 μm behind a shock wave with G_0 at 10.6 μm in a rapid expansion leads to $(G_0)_{50\mu}/(G_0)_{10.6\mu} \simeq 10^{-4}$ and $(G_0)_{22\mu}/(G_0)_{10.6\mu} \simeq 2 \times 10^{-4}$. Clearly, the nonequilibrium region behind a normal shock wave in CO_2–N_2–He mixtures produces a low-gain medium. A more detailed discussion and comparison of these and other laser properties are contained in Anderson *et al.* (1970).

This study indicates that population inversions occur behind a normal shock front strictly owing to translation–vibration and vibration–vibration molecular energy exchanges in CO_2–N_2–He mixtures. However, the laser properties of this shock-induced nonequilibrium flow are clearly not as promising as those of gasdynamic lasers operating on the principle of rapid expansion.

Chapter VII

CO_2–N_2 Gasdynamic Lasers: State-of-the-Art

7.1 Introduction

As described in the previous chapters, the CO_2–N_2–H_2O or He gasdynamic laser (GDL) has spearheaded a breakthrough in high-energy lasers. The high-energy gas laser is clearly a modern reality. Moreover, the technology of these lasers is currently growing in at least three directions, namely, gasdynamic, electric discharge, and chemical lasers.

The basic physical process common to all these lasers is the competition between stimulated emission and absorption of monochromatic radiation, where the radiation (photon) energy corresponds to the difference between two distinct energy levels of an atomic or molecular system. It has been shown in Chapter II that stimulated emission will win over absorption if a population inversion exists between the two energy levels, i.e., if $(N_2 - N_1) > 0$, and therefore laser energy can in principle be extracted from the gas. In electric discharge lasers, the upper energy level is preferentially populated by collisions with electrons energized by an electric field; in chemical lasers, the products of highly energetic chemical reactions are formed directly in vibrationally or electronically excited states with the upper levels preferentially populated; in gasdynamic lasers, an initially hot gas in thermodynamic equilibrium is rapidly expanded through a supersonic nozzle, and an inversion is formed by differential relaxation processes in the nonequilibrium nozzle flow. Of these three types of lasers, the gasdynamic laser has produced the highest continuous wave power to date.

The results embodied in the previous chapters represent (for the most part) a "first generation" of GDL technology, where mixtures of CO_2–N_2–H_2O or He are utilized at typical conditions of $p_0 \simeq 20$ atm, $T_0 \simeq 1200$°K, $h^* \simeq 1$ mm, $A_e/A^* \simeq 20$, and water mole fraction $X_{H_2O} = 0.01$. In light of this previous work, the purpose of the present chapter is twofold: (1) To survey some recent advances contributing to the "second generation" of GDL technology, and (2) to present experimental and theoretical results typifying these advances. In particular, this second generation of GDLs is characterized by higher reservoir temperatures and pressures, smaller nozzle throat heights, larger area ratios, and larger H_2O contents.

As a final introductory note, in the following sections all theoretical values for small-signal gain and maximum available energy are obtained from the time-dependent nonequilibrium nozzle analysis discussed in Chapter IV and are calculated with the computer code described by Glowacki and Anderson (1971). As discussed in Chapter IV, this analysis fully couples the vibrational kinetic rate equations with the governing quasi-one-dimensional flow equations of continuity, momentum, and energy. Nonequilibrium conditions are included both upstream and downstream of the nozzle throat. A simplified vibrational model is used that approximates the detailed molecular energy transfer. The experimental results discussed in Chapter V show that the model and analysis of Chapter IV yield reasonable agreement with experimental data for gasdynamic laser gain. Also in the present discussion, the maximum available energy e_{max} is always the local value at the nozzle exit; hence e_{max} takes into account the vibrational relaxation in the nozzle. In this manner the present e_{max} is different from that defined by Gerry (1970), where the maximum available energy is based on reservoir conditions. The precise definition and calculation of e_{max} is given in Chapter IV.

7.2 Increased H_2O Content

For CO_2–N_2 gasdynamic lasers, the presence of H_2O or He is extremely beneficial for the rapid deactivation of the lower laser level; indeed, such a "catalyst" is necessary for the production of high gain and efficient extraction of laser power. The typical GDL described by Gerry (1970) is combustion-driven, therefore H_2O rather than He is the meaningful catalyst for such devices. Experience with the first generation of GDL technology indicated that gain is a very sensitive function of H_2O content. Along with the beneficial deactivation of the lower level, there is also the competing detrimental deactivation of the upper level due to H_2O. Hence, with the first generation of GDLs, an optimum amount of H_2O in the gas mixture was found to be on the order of 1%, i.e., $X_{H_2O} = 0.01$. For H_2O contents much larger than this, the collisional deactivation of the upper laser level is overwhelming. Such effects are shown by the lower curves in Figs. 7.1 and 7.2. In Figs. 7.1 and 7.2 theoretical values for peak small-signal gain and maximum available energy, respectively, are given as a function of X_{H_2O}. (In the spirit of the SI system of units, e_{max} is given in kilojoules per kilogram; however, the more common GDL unit is kilojoules per pound$_m$, where 1 kJ/lb$_m$ = 2.2 kJ/kg.) The lower curves in both these figures typify the first-generation technology, for which the maximum peak gain is clearly seen to occur around $X_{H_2O} = 0.01$.

The low value of $X_{H_2O} \simeq 0.01$ for optimum gain places a severe constraint on candidate fuels for GDLs. Most conventional fuel–oxidizer combinations producing CO_2 and N_2 also produce H_2O far in excess of 1%. (Pallay and

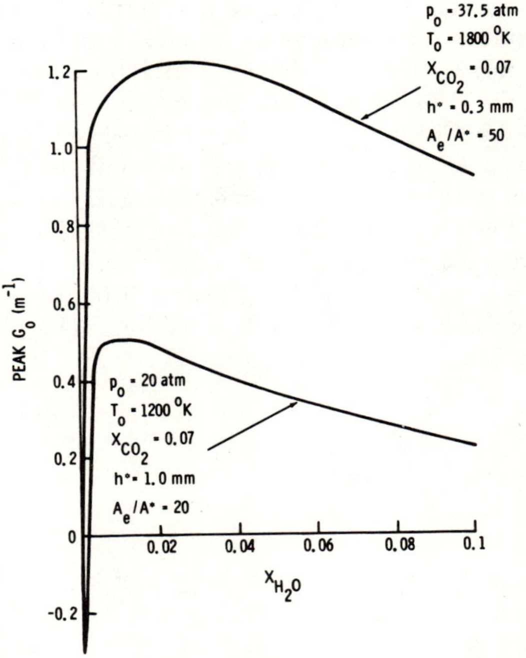

FIG. 7.1 Peak gain as a function of H_2O content for first- and second-generation gasdynamic lasers. (After Anderson and Harris, 1972a.)

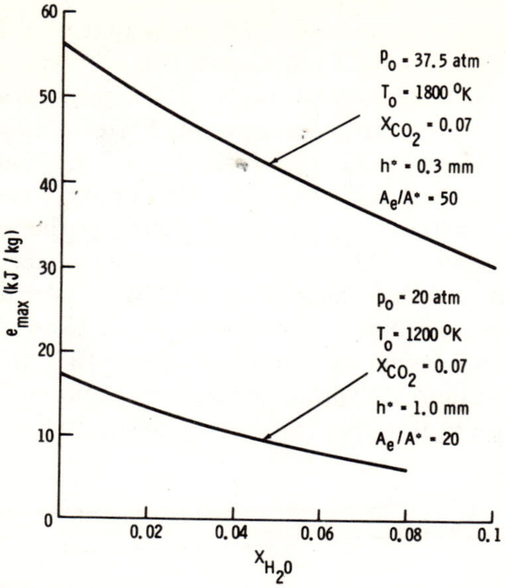

FIG. 7.2 Maximum available laser energy as a function of H_2O content for first- and second-generation gasdynamic lasers.

Zovko, 1973). Therefore, recent efforts have been made to study the effects of higher H_2O content on GDLs, say, in the range from 1 to 10%. In this vein Yatsiv *et al.* (1971) and Tulip and Seguin (1971) have operated GDLs with attendant H_2O contents up to 8%. (Tulip and Seguin have recently used gasoline in a GDL.) Also, some earlier gain measurements made in the NOL 3-MW arc tunnel covered a H_2O range from 0 to 6%. These experiments have shown that small-signal gain does indeed persist at high H_2O content. This is also clearly shown by the lower curve of Fig. 7.1, where G_0 persists for H_2O content at least as high as 10%, albeit substantially reduced from its optimum value, which occurs around 1%. Of more consequence for first-generation GDLs, however, is the drastic reduction of e_{max} shown in the lower curve of Fig. 7.2 for higher H_2O content. Therefore, we are led to the conclusion that, for the h^*, T_0, p_0, and A_e/A^* characteristics of first-generation technology, GDLs *can* operate with high H_2O content but with severe penalities in efficiency. That is, the percentage loss in G_0 and e_{max} is very large as X_{H_2O} is increased from 0.01 to 0.1.

On the other hand, high values of X_{H_2O} appear to be more compatible with second-generation technology (lower h^*, higher T_0, p_0, and A_e/A^*). This is clearly shown by the upper curves of Figs. 7.1 and 7.2, which typify this newer technology. For $A_e/A^* = 50$, $h^* = 0.3$ mm, and $T_0 = 1800$°K, the theoretical results shown in Fig. 7.1 imply that peak gain is maximum for $X_{H_2O} = 0.025$ and that this maximum is fairly flat for X_{H_2O} from 0.01 to 0.06. Indeed, a more detailed study of the theoretical results reveals that, for the stronger expansions associated with the second-generation nozzles, the lower laser level as well as the upper level tends to freeze inside the nozzle. Hence, more H_2O is necessary to promote rapid equilibration of the lower level with the translational energy of the gas. This effect is shown in Fig. 7.3, which illustrates the variations of the upper and lower laser level vibrational temperatures T_{001} and T_{100}, respectively, as a function of distance for several different values of X_{H_2O}. Note that, for $X_{H_2O} = 0.01$, the lower level is far from equilibrated and that values on the order of $X_{H_2O} = 0.04$ are needed to promote rapid equilibration. Therefore, we are

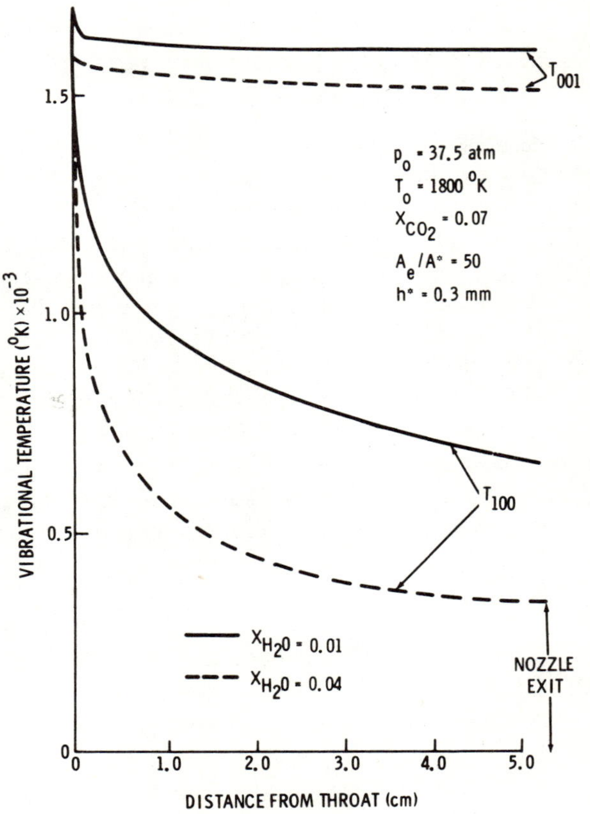

FIG. 7.3 Vibrational temperature distributions inside the nozzle for different values of X_{H_2O}.

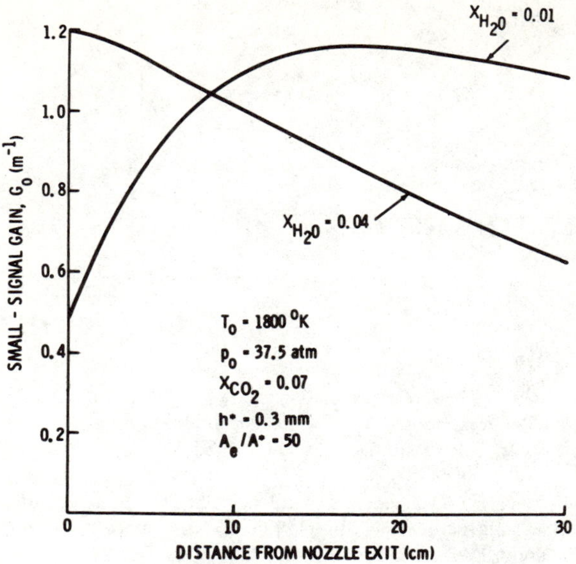

FIG. 7.4 Small-signal gain distributions downstream of the nozzle exit for two different values of X_{H_2O}.

led to conclude that second-generation GDLs are more amenable to higher H_2O content and that a wider range of fuels for GDLs is now a possibility.

The gain profiles are markedly different between high and low H_2O content. This is shown in Fig. 7.4, where G_0 is given as a function of distance downstream of the nozzle exit. In comparison to the case for $X_{H_2O} = 0.01$, note in Fig. 7.4 that the peak G_0 for $X_{H_2O} = 0.04$ occurs nearer the nozzle exit and that gain drops off more rapidly with distance. This implies a constraint on the laser cavity design for mixtures with high H_2O content, namely, that power has to be extracted in shorter distances. However, such rapid power extraction appears feasible, for example, with an unstable resonator, as described by Gerry (1970) and as discussed in Chapter X.

The results shown in Figs. 7.1–7.4 are theoretical and may be a bit optimistic. The kinetic rates embodied in these results are obtained from Taylor and Bitterman (1967), with the lower laser level deactivation rate due to H_2O modified to account for the calculations of Sharma (1971). (See Chapter V.) They do not include the updated rates described in Appendixes A and B of the present book. The effect of the newer rates on such calculations, along with a comparison with the experimental data of Vamos (1974), is shown in Figs. 7.5 and 7.6. Vamos has conducted a systematic series of shock tunnel tests covering first-generation (Fig. 7.5) GDLs (20:1 nozzle area ratio) as well as second-generation (Fig.

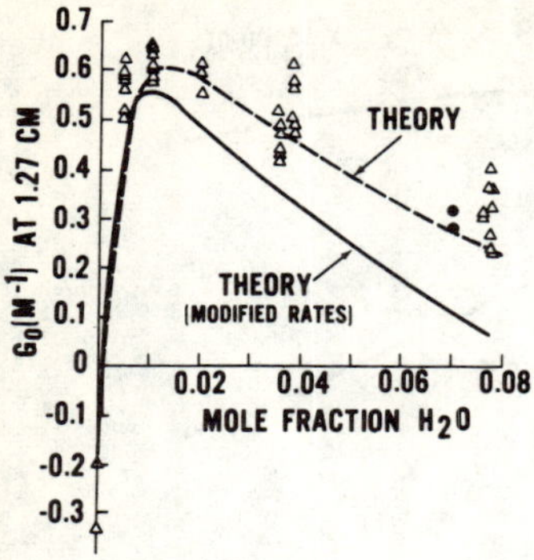

FIG. 7.5

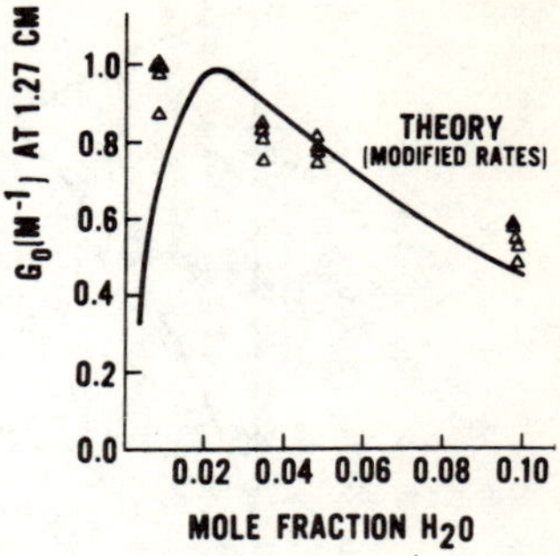

FIG. 7.6

FIG. 7.5 Effect of H_2O content on small-signal gain. Location is 1.27 cm downstream of the nozzle exit. Gas mixture has 7% CO_2 constant. First-generation gasdynamic laser with 20:1 area ratio nozzle. 1 mm throat height, $T_0 = 1800°K$, $p_0 = 20$ atm. (After Vamos, 1974.)

FIG. 7.6 Effect of H_2O content on small-signal gain for a second-generation gasdynamic laser. Location, percentage of CO_2, and T_0 same as in Fig. 7.5. $p_0 = 37.5$ atm; 0.37 mm throat height. (After Vamos, 1974.)

7.6) GDLs (50:1 nozzle area ratio). In both figures the theoretical and experimental results for small-signal gain show that G_0 persists at high H_2O content. Therefore, even though the results of Figs. 7.1–7.4 may be slightly optimistic, the trends and conclusions shown are still valid.

7.3 Increased Temperature

The obvious advantage of increasing the reservoir temperature T_0 of GDLs is that the reservoir vibrational energy per unit mass increases. On the other hand, a disadvantage of increasing T_0 is that collisional deactivation becomes more rapid, and therefore not all of the increased reservoir vibrational energy is realized at the nozzle exit. Another disadvantage is increased heating of GDL components. However, increasing T_0 is certainly a viable means of increasing output power per unit mass flow, and high temperatures are therefore a major characteristic of second-generation GDLs. Because the nozzle exit temperature should be low ($T_{exit} \simeq 300°K$) in order to keep the lower laser level population low, increasing T_0 automatically implies increasing A_e/A^*. For GDLs that exhaust to the atmosphere with a fixed diffuser efficiency, this also automatically implies increasing p_0. Therefore, in light of the above discussion, the reasons are clear

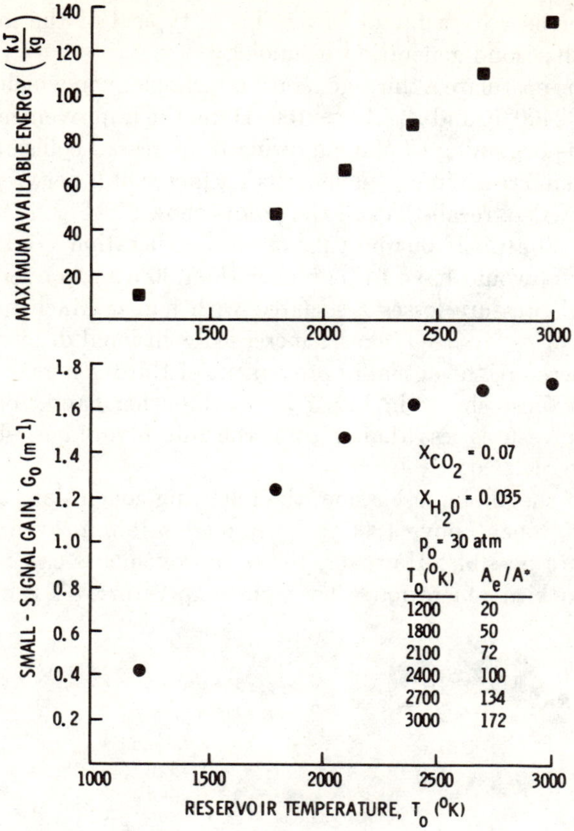

FIG. 7.7 Effect of increasing reservoir temperature on peak gain and maximum available energy. (After Anderson and Harris, 1972a.)

for choosing the conditions that contrast the first- and second-generation technology in both Figs. 7.1 and 7.2.

The purpose of this section is to discuss the results of a numerical experiment indicating the advantages of increasing T_0. These results are shown in Fig. 7.7, where G_0 and e_{max} are plotted versus T_0. For each numerical point shown, A_e/A^* is different. The area ratio is increased as T_0 increases in order to maintain $T_{exit} \simeq 300°K$. For the sake of consistency, the reservoir pressure is held fixed at 30 atm for these points; i.e., the GDL is assumed to exhaust to a variable back pressure generally less than 1 atm.

Examining Fig. 7.7, the improvements brought about by increasing T_0 from 1200 to 1800°K are clearly seen. Peak G_0 is dramatically enhanced, and e_{max} increases by a factor of 5. This is typical of the improvements incurred with second-generation technology.

Now, let us postulate a third-generation technology in which T_0 is further increased to 2400°K and $A_e/A^* \simeq 100$. Here, the improvements are not so striking. G_0 is beginning to plateau owing to increased collisional deactivation, and the increase in e_{max} is less than a factor of 2 between $T_0 = 1800$ and 2400°K. Also, recall that all the points shown in Fig. 7.7 are for $p_0 =$ constant $= 30$ atm. If our postulated third-generation GDL exhausts to 1 atm, then p_0 would have to be higher than 30 atm to overcome the increased total pressure losses associated with higher Mach number flows. An increase in p_0, by itself, causes increased collisional deactivation in the flow, and therefore the actual improvement of third-generation GDLs will be less than those shown in Fig. 7.7. On the other hand, for GDLs that exhaust to pressures less than 1 atm, the full advantages shown in Fig. 7.7 might be realized.

In light of the above discussion, the following conclusions are made. By increasing T_0 much above 1800°K, only moderate improvements (factors of 2 or 3) are possible. However, these improvements can be important. Therefore, a third-generation, very high temperature GDL may be worth

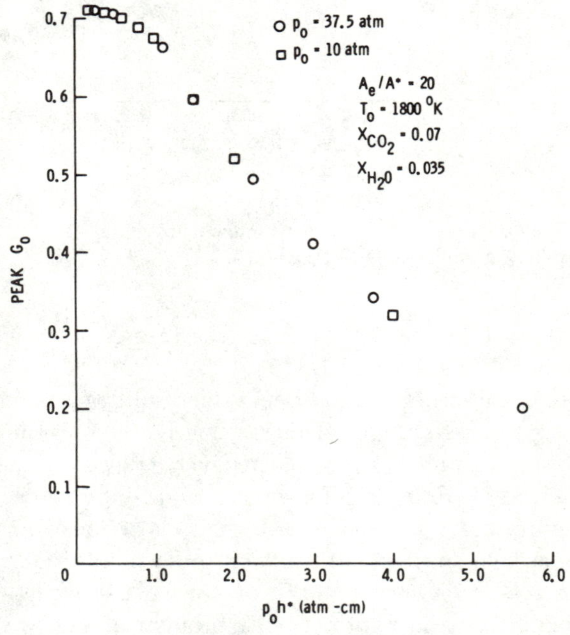

FIG. 7.8 Binary scaling of small-signal gain for a low area ratio nozzle.

further consideration. In the process many important questions will have to be answered: for example, are there appropriate fuels that yield a 3000°K combustion temperature, and how difficult will it be to maintain the critical elements of GDL hardware at these temperatures?

7.4 Binary Scaling

Gerry (1970) and Greenberg *et al.* (1970) have pointed out that current GDLs can be scaled according to the parameter p_0h^*. This is anticipated

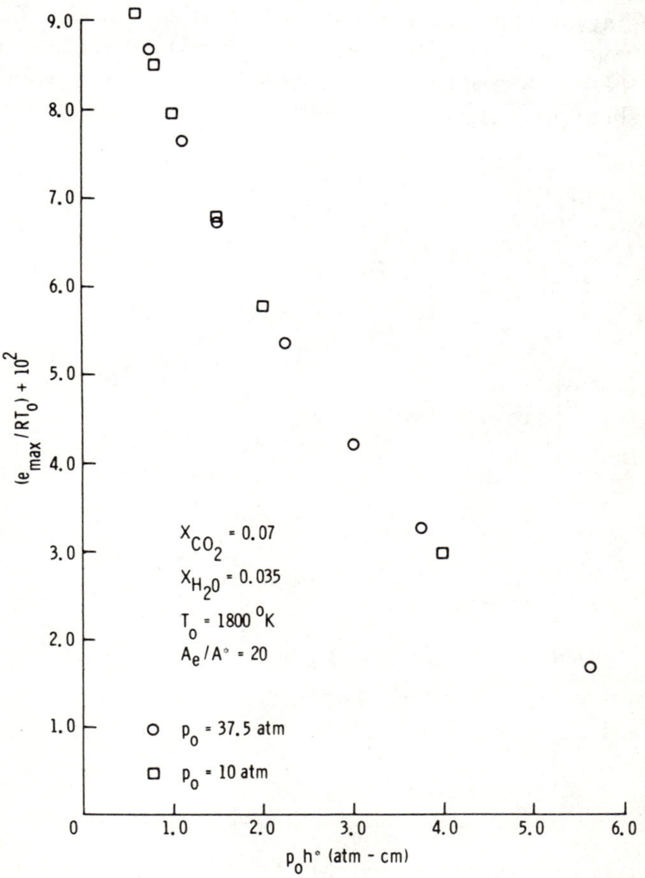

FIG. 7.9 Binary scaling of maximum available energy for a low area ratio nozzle.

because two-body collisional deactivation dominates the kinetics. The purpose of this section is to examine in more detail the implications of binary scaling on GDL flows.

Figures 7.8 and 7.9 contain numerical results for peak G_0 and e_{max}, respectively, plotted versus p_0h^* for a set of GDL nozzle flows with the same mixture ratio, nozzle contour, T_0, and $A_e/A^* = 20$. Figures 7.10 and 7.11 contain similar results, except that $A_e/A^* = 50$. In each figure only p_0 and h^* are varied as shown. Clearly, the peak G_0 and e_{max} are unique functions of the p_0h^* product, thus explicitly demonstrating the binary scaling. In addition, several trends are important to note, as follows.

(1) The variation of G_0 and e_{max} with p_0h^* is not linear; i.e., halving the p_0h^* does not necessarily double the gain or e_{max}. This is particularly true for G_0 at low values of $p_0h^* < 1$ atm-cm, as seen in Figs. 7.8 and 7.10.

(2) Figures 7.8 and 7.10 show that $p_0h^* \simeq 1$ atm-cm is a reasonable value of the binary scaling parameter for high gain. This value has been stated earlier by Greenberg *et al.* (1970). In the same vein, Gerry (1970)

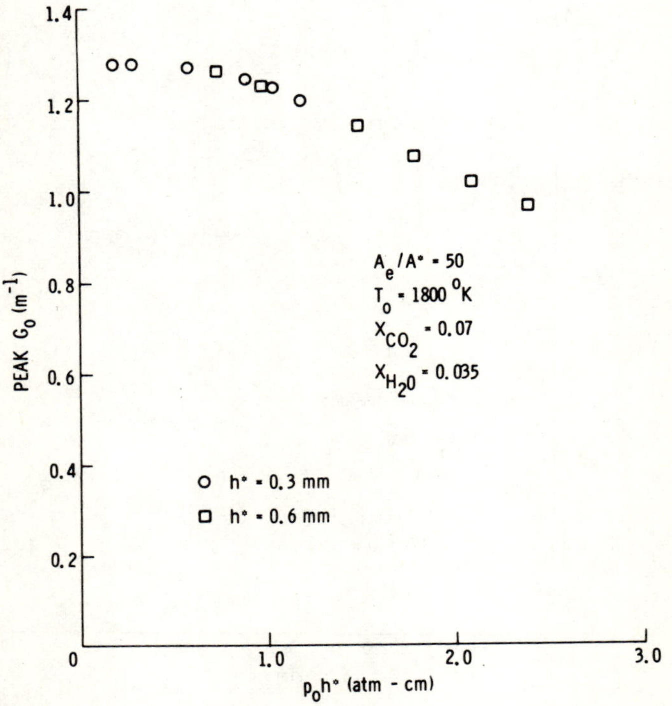

FIG. 7.10 Binary scaling of small-signal gain for a high area ratio nozzle.

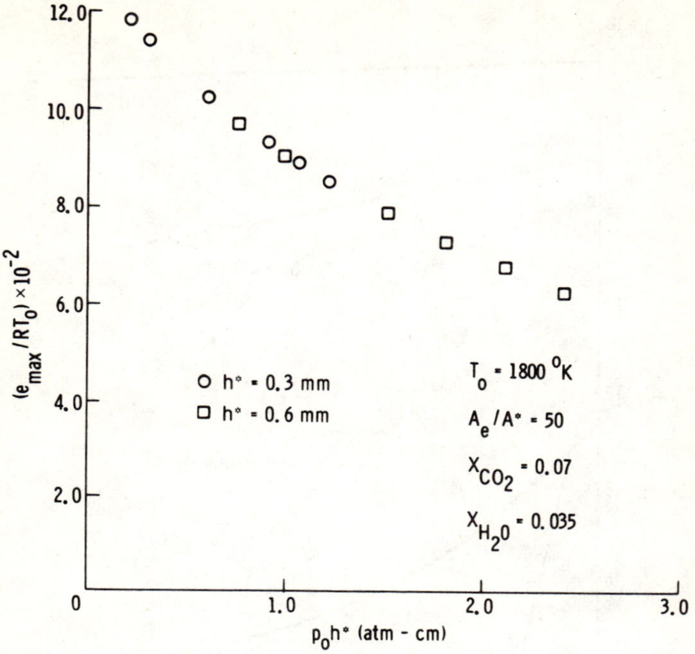

FIG. 7.11 Binary scaling of maximum available energy for a high area ratio nozzle.

has pointed out a criterion for adequate freezing of the nozzle flow, namely, that $p_0h^* < 2(p\tau_{eff})_{T^*}u^*$ This criterion is simply a statement that, in the throat region, the flow residence time h^*/u^* should be less than the effective relaxation time $(p\tau_{eff})_{T^*}/p^* \approx (p\tau_{eff})_{T^*}/0.5p_0$. For the flow conditions in Figs. 7.8–7.11, $2(p\tau_{eff})_{T^*}u^* \simeq 1.25$ atm-cm; hence, a value of $p_0h^* \simeq 1$ atm-cm satisfies the above criterion.

(3) Major increases in G_0 cannot be obtained by reducing p_0h^* below 1 atm-cm. This is clearly seen in Figs. 7.8 and 7.10, where G_0 essentially reaches a plateau for $p_0h^* < 1$ atm-cm. The basic reason for this behavior is that, for low values of p_0h^*, *both* the upper and lower laser levels tend to freeze in the nozzle expansion. In fact, in the theoretical limit of $p_0 = 0$, hence $p_0h^* = 0$, both the upper and lower laser levels would freeze at their equilibrium reservoir values, no population inversion would exist anywhere in the flow, the gain would be negative, and e_{max} would be zero. These trends are illustrated in Fig. 7.12, which gives the vibrational and translational temperatures for $p_0h^* = 0.21$ atm-cm (solid lines) and 1.2 atm-cm (dashed lines) as a function of distance from the nozzle exit. First, consider the solid lines. For $p_0h^* = 0.21$ atm-cm, the tendency for T_{100} to "hang up"

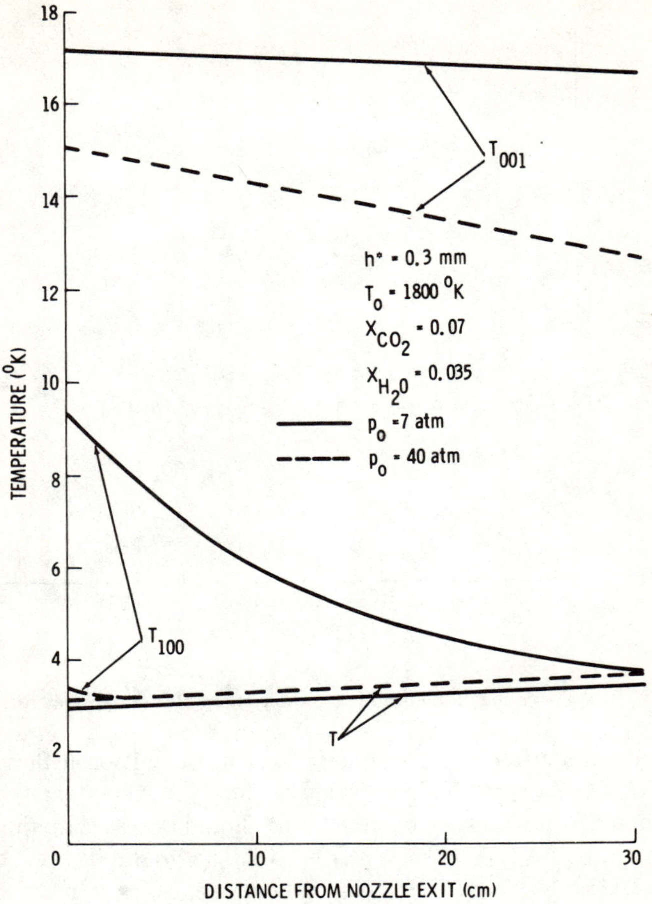

FIG. 7.12 Vibrational and static temperature distributions downstream of the nozzle exit for two different values of p_0. $A_e/A^* = 50$.

is quite evident. Indeed, a downstream distance of more than 30 cm is required before T_{100} equilibrates with T. At 30 cm the peak gain of 1.28 m^{-1} is finally achieved. In comparison consider the dotted lines for $p_0h^* = 1.2$ atm-cm. The upper level vibrational temperature T_{001} is less than the previous case; by itself, this will reduce G_0. However, T_{100} has relaxed quite rapidly and is essentially equilibrated near the nozzle exit; this will favor the gain. For this case a peak G_0 of 1.2 m^{-1} is achieved near the nozzle exit.

With these trends in mind, there appears to be little benefit in striving for *exceptionally* small values of $p_0 h^*$ in gasdynamic lasers. Indeed, it appears to be sufficient to satisfy the criterion, $p_0 h^* < 2(p\tau_{eff})_T{}^* u^*$.

7.5 Fuels for Gasdynamic Lasers

The conventional gasdynamic laser is a somewhat "touchy" device with regard to optimum operating conditions; the equilibrium reservoir mixture ratio of CO_2, N_2, H_2O, or He, the pressure and temperature of the reservoir gas, the size and area ratio of the nozzles, and the optical design of the laser cavity all exert first-order influence on power output. Moreover, the allowable latitude in some of these quantities is very narrow; the previous discussion on the effect of H_2O content is a case in point. If the reservoir conditions are obtained in an arc tunnel or shock tunnel as described in Chapter V, then optimum conditions for mixture ratio, pressure, and temperature can be almost simultaneously achieved because these quantities can be varied rather independently of each other in such laboratory devices. However, for gasdynamic lasers operating outside of the laboratory environment for various military or industrial purposes, the reservoir gas must be obtained in a more self-contained fashion. To date, the only such fashion has been chemical combustion; indeed, many existing GDLs are first cousins to rocket engines. Figure 1.2 of Chapter I shows a photograph of a combustion-driven GDL. Unfortunately, the mixture ratio of the combustion products and the reservoir temperature and pressure are no longer independent of each other for such combustion-driven GDLs. Hence, the problem of obtaining optimum operating conditions is greatly compounded. The purpose of this section is to describe this problem and to discuss some of the solutions already in practice as well as some that have promise for the future.

An excellent review of fuels, oxidizers, and gas generators for combustion-driven gasdynamic lasers is given by Pallay and Zovko (1973), from which much of the data of this section is obtained.

For the gasdynamic laser, a self-contained fuel–oxidizer combination must provide equilibrium combustion products with the proper ratio of $CO_2/N_2/H_2O$ at pressures and temperatures compatible with reasonably efficient operation. Conventional hydrocarbon rocket fuels produce CO_2, N_2, and H_2O, but unfortunately not in ratios even remotely approaching the 10%/89%/1% mixtures typical of our discussions in the previous chapters. Most rocket fuels yield far too much H_2O and CO_2, and not enough N_2. As a result, the first generation of combustion-driven GDLs

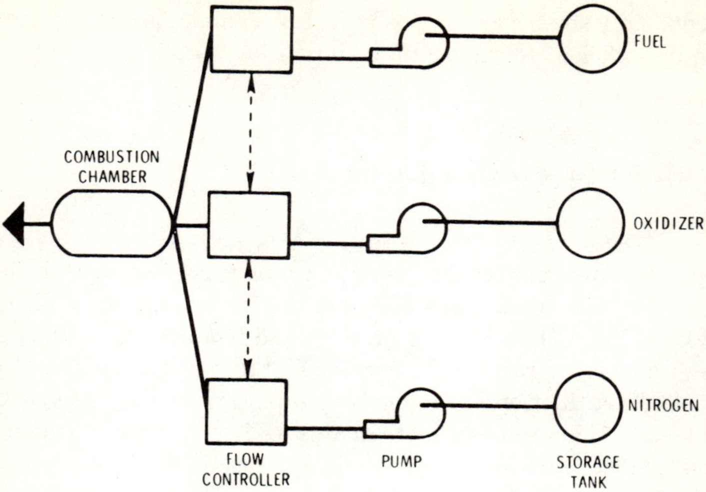

FIG. 7.13 Bipropellant gas generator with N_2 diluent. (After Pallay and Zovko, 1973.)

has burned carbon monoxide in either air or oxygen to form CO_2 with an auxiliary source of N_2 mixed with the combustion products and a dash of CH_4 or H_2 added to form H_2O. This type of system is shown schematically in Fig. 7.13, taken from the work of Pallay and Zovko (1973). In this system, the fuel, CO, and oxidizer, O_2 or air, are pumped into a combustion chamber where CO_2 is formed by the reaction $CO + \frac{1}{2}O_2 \rightarrow CO_2$. The combustion is usually initiated by a spark or other ignitor; the reaction is not hypergolic. Nitrogen is added as a diluent in an amount sufficient to obtain the desired CO_2/N_2 ratio. Also, small amounts of CH_4 or H_2 are added to form the proper amount of water vapor via the reaction $CH_4 + O_2 \rightarrow 2H_2O + C$ or $H_2 + \frac{1}{2}O_2 \rightarrow H_2O$. In this fashion, the $CO_2/N_2/H_2O$ mixture ratio can be tailored as desired; however, the reservoir temperature is a function of this ratio and increases as the amount of CO_2 in the combustion products increases.

This bipropellant system of CO–O_2 or air is reasonably convenient and well understood, hence explaining its use in the first generation of gasdynamic lasers. However, thermodynamically it is inferior to a number of other possible fuel–ozidizer combinations. To see this more clearly, a comparison of the heat released by several combinations yielding CO_2 as a combustion product is made in Table 7.1. Here, eight different fuels, burning with either O_2 or N_2O, are compared on the basis of heat output. Clearly CO is the *least* energetic fuel. Also, examining Table 7.1, N_2O is seen to be a more effective oxidizer than O_2, oxidizers in the gaseous state

TABLE 7.1

Comparison of Heat Outputs of Several Carbon Dioxide Producing Fuels[a]

Oxidizer Fuel	Oxygen[b] (gaseous)	Oxygen[b] (liquid)	Nitrous Oxide[b] (gaseous)	Nitrous Oxide[b] (liquid)	Toxocity
CO (gaseous)	67.6	66.1	87.2	82.3	high
C (solid)	94.1	91.0	133.3	—	none
C_3O_2 (gaseous)	86.7	84.5	112.7	106.2	high (?)
C_2N_2 (liquid)	128.2	125.1	167.4	157.6	high
C_2N_2 (gaseous)	131.0	127.9	170.2	160.4	high
C_6H_6 (liquid)	124.8	121.2	171.4	159.9	low
C_5H_5N (liquid)	126.1	122.5	172.7	161.2	low
C_7H_5N (liquid)	119.5	116.2	163.5	152.7	high

[a] After Pallay and Zovko (1973).
[b] Heat released in kcal/mole CO_2.

yield more heat than in the liquid state (obviously due to the heat of vaporization), and the hydrocarbons, such as benzene (C_6H_6), are considerably more energetic than CO. This comparison points the way to more advanced fuels for second- and third-generation GDLs. For example, let us single out the benzene–nitrous oxide combination. Benzene is an attractive fuel because it leads to higher combustion temperatures and its handling properties are similar to gasoline—it is a *practical* fuel and reasonably safe. Nitrous oxide (N_2O) is a liquid at room temperature and 50 atm, hence it is relatively easy to store. It also has a high nitrogen content. Recent experiments have shown that combustion of C_6H_6 with N_2O is almost soot free; this is a necessity for efficient laser action, since solid particles in the laser gas will scatter radiation and hence attenuate the laser beam. Also, note that C_6H_6 combustion will yield CO_2 and H_2O in a ratio of 2:1. This is the motivation for the 7% CO_2/3.5% H_2O mixture chosen for the calculations shown in Figs. 7.7–7.12.

The dependence of the reservoir temperature on the CO_2 concentration of the products of combustion is clearly shown in Fig. 7.14, which further compares benzene with carbon monoxide as fuels for combustion with both O_2 and N_2O as oxidizers. This is an important figure. For example, it shows that

(a) Benzene and nitrous oxide combustion yields by far the highest reservoir temperature over the range of CO_2 concentration from 7 to 15%—the range of interest for conventional GDLs.

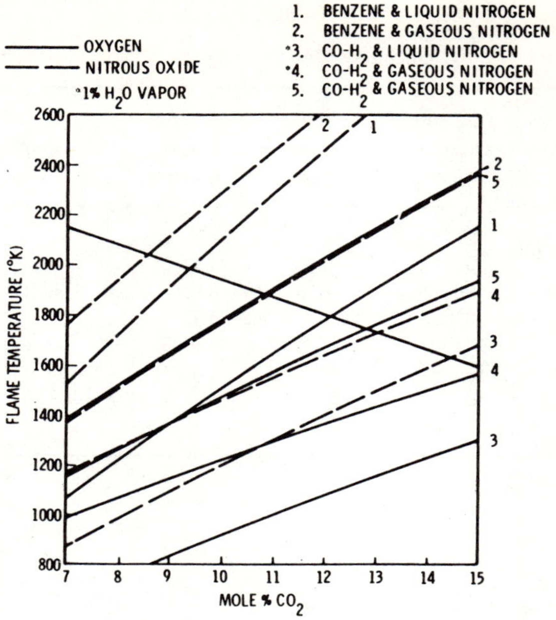

FIG. 7.14 Flame temperature as a function of CO_2 content for different gasdynamic laser fuel–oxidizer combinations. (After Pallay and Zovko, 1973.)

(b) For any of the given fuel–oxidizer combinations, the reservoir temperature increases as the CO_2 concentration increases. In other words, the mixture ratio and reservoir temperature are *not* independent parameters, contrary to the situation in an arc tunnel or shock tunnel.

(c) The intersection of curve 2 for C_6H_6–N_2O with the ordinate shows that a relatively high temperature of approximately 1800°K can be obtained with the formation of only 7% CO_2 (and consequently 3.5% H_2O). These are precisely the reservoir conditions chosen for the calculations shown in Figs. 7.8–7.12.

(d) Reservoir temperatures associated with first-generation GDLs ($T_0 \approx 1200$°K) are readily obtained with CO–O_2 combustion. However, temperatures associated with second-generation GDLs ($T_0 \approx 1800$°K) have to be obtained by either burning CO with N_2O with attendant CO_2 concentrations above 11%, or by burning C_6H_6 with N_2O producing lower CO_2 concentrations (around 7%).

In summary, CO burning in O_2 or air has been used successfully in first-generation GDLs, and CO burning in N_2O is feasible for second-generation devices. In both these combinations, the H_2O content is supplied separately and independently by burning small amounts of CH_4 or H_2. Another viable combination for second-generation GDLs is C_6H_6 burning in N_2O, which automatically supplies a CO_2/H_2O ratio of 2:1. To date C_6H_6–N_2O combustion has been successfully examined in the laboratory, but it is too new to have yet found application in practical GDLs.

There are other fuel–oxidizer combinations that are possible, as evident from Table 7.1. However, a number of these combinations pose safety problems associated with high toxicity. Even CO is guilty on this count, whereas C_6H_6 is much safer. However, solid carbon has no toxicity and does provide a substantial increase in heat output compared to CO. For this reason, C (solid) has attracted some attention as a fuel for gasdynamic lasers. A method for burning carbon has been suggested by Pallay and Zovko (1973), wherein a carbon matrix is preheated after which air is flowed through the matrix. This is shown schematically in Fig. 7.15. The O_2 in the air reacts with the carbon, but because of the high surface area of the carbon, CO rather than CO_2 is the dominant combustion product. The products CO and N_2 then flow at temperature $T1$ into a second combustion chamber where more air is added to form CO_2 from the incoming CO. The final products of combustion are CO_2 and N_2 at temperature $T2$. The temperatures $T1$ and $T2$ are shown in Fig. 7.16 as a function of final CO_2 concentration. Note that this scheme can produce the high temperatures associated with second-generation GDLs but with higher attendant CO_2 concentrations (above 13%) than either CO or C_6H_6 burning in N_2O. (A relatively high CO_2 concentration is not altogether bad; indeed, Eq. (2.20) indicates that, everything else being equal,

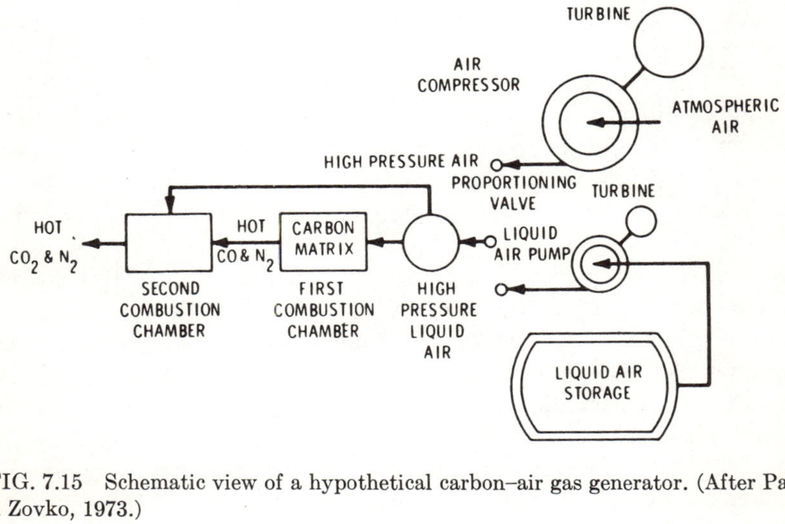

FIG. 7.15 Schematic view of a hypothetical carbon–air gas generator. (After Pallay and Zovko, 1973.)

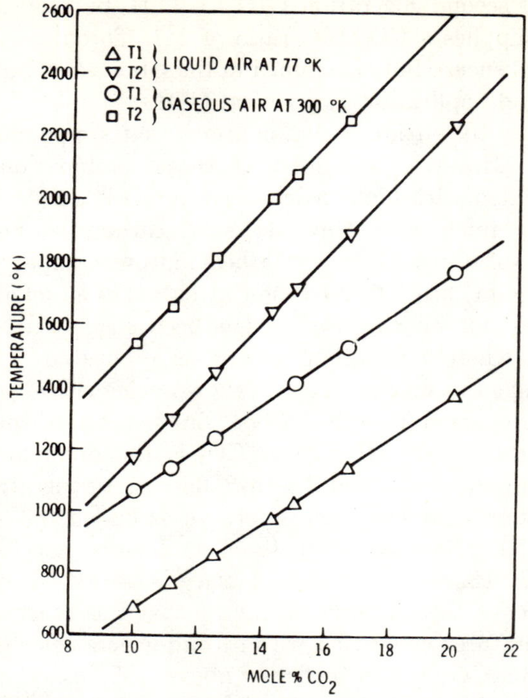

FIG. 7.16 Theoretical gas temperature as a function of CO_2 content for the carbon–air combustor. (After Pallay and Zovko, 1973.)

small-signal gain G_0 is directly proportional to the CO_2 concentration. However, everything else is not equal, because CO_2 increases the rate of vibrational deactivation of the upper level via the reactions given by Eqs. (3.11) and (3.13); i.e., the actual population inversion created by the nonequilibrium nozzle expansion is adversely affected if too much CO_2 is present in the gas. Hence, the proper amount of CO_2 for a GDL mixture is a compromise, and optimum amounts usually fall somewhere between the extremes of 1 and 20%, depending on conditions of p_0, T_0, and nozzle size.)

Referring back to Fig. 7.7, a possible third-generation GDL incorporating temperatures as high as 3000°K was discussed. However, Figs. 7.14 and 7.16 show that producing such high temperatures by chemical combustion while at the same time keeping the CO_2 concentrations at relatively low values is not easy. In fact, by themselves, the fuel–oxidizer combinations discussed so far are not sufficient. However, the calculations shown in Figs. 7.14 and 7.16 assume that the gaseous nitrogen or air is pumped into the combustion chamber at room temperature. Instead, if the diluent were *preheated* to above 1000°K before being pumped into the combustion chamber, then considerably higher reservoir temperatures than shown in Figs. 7.14 and 7.16 would be possible. This leads to a consideration of hot nitrogen generators for possible use in gasdynamic lasers.

A scheme for such a generator is described by Pallay and Zovko (1973). It consists of burning sodium azide (NaN_3) with N_2O to form the equilibrium products shown in Table 7.2. Note that, for the very fuel-rich case (composition 2), 99.2% of the products is N_2 at 1006°K. For composition 1, 92.8% N_2 is formed at a higher temperature of 1236°K. These mixtures appear to be good sources of hot N_2 for use as a diluent in gasdynamic lasers. However, there may be one drawback. These mixtures also contain gaseous sodium, Na. The calculations of Fisher and Smith (1970) indicate that Na acting as a collision partner with vibrationally excited N_2 will cause a very rapid T–V deactivation of the N_2 via the reaction given by Eq. (3.11). In fact, their calculations show rate constants reflecting N_2 vibrational deactivation by Na that is orders of magnitude faster than any other species in the gas. Therefore, the presence of Na in GDL mixtures may be extremely deleterious to gain and power. This fact is reinforced by the results of Anderson (1972a), who modified the time-dependent GDL analysis described in Chapter IV to take into account the effect of Na.

TABLE 7.2

Theoretically Computed Compositions of Reaction Products Resulting from Sodium and Nitrous Oxide[a]

Reactants	Composition 1	Composition 2
Sodium azide (NaN_3)	90% (weight)	95% (weight)
Nitrous oxide (N_2O)	10% (weight)	5% (weight)
Pressure	400 psia	400 psia
Temperature of products	1236°K	1006°K
Gaseous reaction products[b]		
Nitrogen (M_2)	92.8% (mole)	99.2% (mole)
Sodium (Na)	5.9	0.7
Sodium (Na_2)	1.3	0.1
Liquid and solid reaction products[c]		
Sodium (Na)	16.5% (weight)	27.9% (weight)
Sodium Oxide (NaiO)	13.4	6.7

[a] After Pallay and Zovko (1973).

[b] Gaseous product compositions are given as mole percent of gaseous product.

[c] Weight percents are based on total product weight.

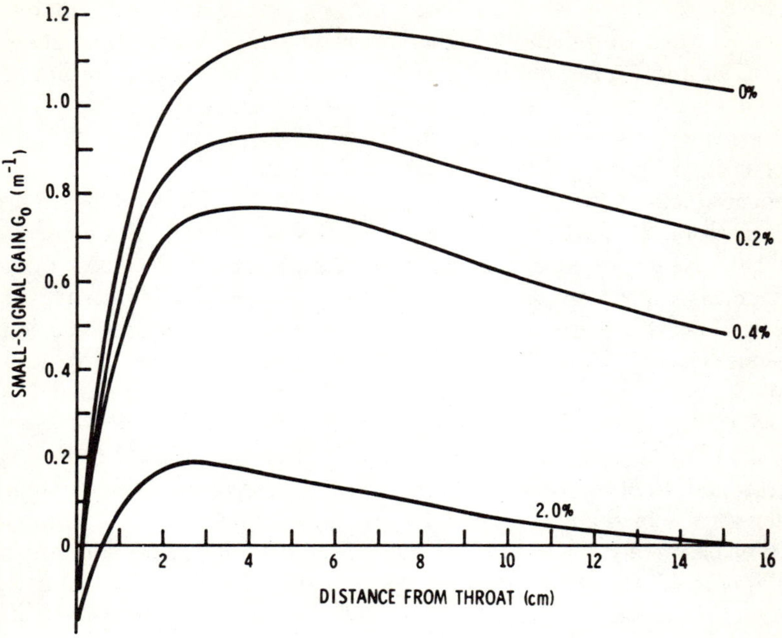

FIG. 7.17 Small-signal gain profiles for different Na contents from 0 to 2%. T_0 = 1600°K; p_0 = 37.5 atm; A/A^* = 50; h^* = 0.3 mm; X_{CO_2} = 0.07; X_{H_2O} = 0.035. (After Anderson, 1972a.)

Some results of this study are shown in Fig. 7.17. In this figure, small-signal gain profiles are shown with Na content as a parameter. A serious degradation of gain is shown even with very small amounts of Na. In fact, with 2% Na in the mixture, gain is almost destroyed. These results should not be taken as definitive because they use a *calculated* value for the Na–N_2 rate constant obtained from Fisher and Smith (1970). Calculations of any rate constant are always tenuous and could be in error by an order of magnitude or more. Hence, the study of Anderson (1972a) needs to be confirmed by experiment. However, until such confirmation is achieved, the results shown in Fig. 7.17 serve to temper the use of NaN_3 as a hot N_2 source for gasdynamic lasers.

An alternative source of hot N_2 is suggested by Pallay and Zovko (1973). This is the use of a fixed and/or fluidized bed of iron particles shown in Fig. 7.18. Here, the bed is preheated, and a cold mixture of N_2 and O_2 (air) at temperature T_0 is fed into the inlet. The iron reacts with the O_2,

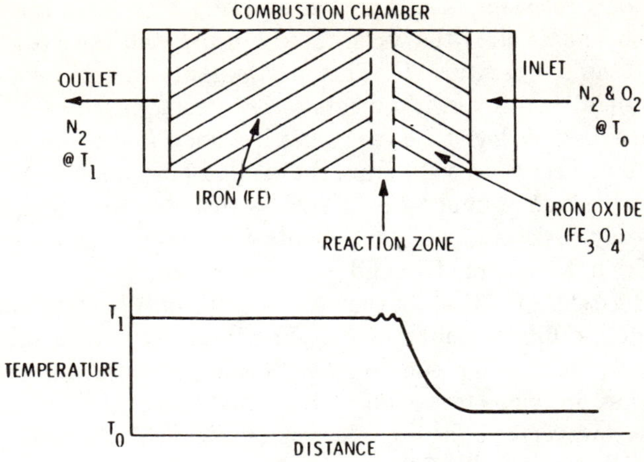

FIG. 7.18 Fixed bed iron–air burner with ignition at inlet and bed preheated. (After Pallay and Zovko, 1973.)

TABLE 7.3

Theoretical Computer Reaction Products from a Solid Propellant Combination[a]

Reactants		Gaseous reaction products		
Ingredient	Weight (grams)	Ingredient	Mole %	Moles
NaN_3	60.08	N_2	72.78	1.533
S	14.82	CO_2	8.68	0.183
C	3.47	NaOH	5.73	0.121
$NaNO_3$	16.55	CO	5.01	0.106
SiO_2	2.00	Na	4.03	0.085
NH_4NO_3	4.00	SO_2	1.67	0.035
		H_2O	1.64	0.035
		H_2	1.95	0.004
		SO	1.04	0.002
Combustion chamber pressure	Adiabatic flame temperature	Solid or liquid reaction products, moles		
(psia)	(°K)	Na_2S (liquid)		Na_2SiO_3 (liqud)
400	2102	.422		.0333

[a] After Pallay and Zovko (1973).

forming Fe_3O_4, releasing heat, and consequently increasing the N_2 temperature. At the outlet all of the O_2 has been burned, and the gas is essentially pure hot N_2 at temperature T_1. This idea is new and has not yet been examined in detail; however, it appears to have some promise.

There are distinct logistic advantages if a solid fuel could be developed for gasdynamic lasers—a solid grain that would burn and produce the right mixture at the right temperature. Work is just starting along these lines. Unfortunately, existing solid propellants for rocket engines produce too much H_2O, not enough N_2, and substantial amounts of CO. Indeed, Pallay and Zovko (1973) state that NaN_3 is the only known solid that can produce the required amount of N_2. When burned with a mix of sulfur, carbon, and other solid compounds, NaN_3 produces gaseous reaction products that are close to a viable GDL mixture. Such a case is given in Table 7.3. However, once again reflecting on Fig. 7.17, the 4.03% Na in the reaction products in Table 7.3 may not be acceptable.

The use of near conventional rocket engine solid propellents for GDLs has recently been given a boost by the results of Vamos (1974) and Tennant *et al.* (1974). These experimental shock tunnel investigations have shown that reasonable small-signal gain is obtainable in GDL mixtures with high CO content. It appears that CO plays much the same role as N_2 in pumping the upper laser level of CO_2. Some typical results from Vamos (1974) are shown in Fig. 7.19. There is an almost linear degradation in gain as the CO content is increased; however, substantial gain still exists even when the N_2 is *completely* replaced by CO. Hence, solid propellants that do not produce "enough" N_2 but that produce substantial amounts of CO may hold some promise for application to gasdynamic lasers.

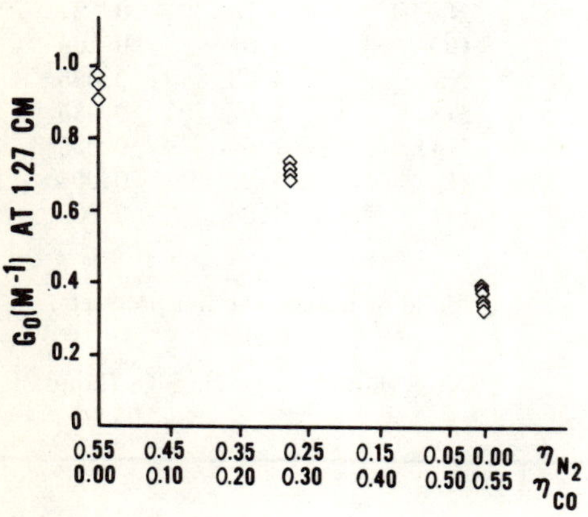

FIG. 7.19 Shock tunnel data for the variation of small-signal gain with CO content from 0 to 55% (total replacement of N_2). (After Vamos, 1974.)

In summary, fuels for combustion-driven gasdynamic lasers are evolving rapidly. The $CO–O_2$ system has been in common use, but other possibilities exist, as described above. In fact, as new generations of high performance GDLs are developed, new fuel–oxidizer combinations and innovative ideas will be absolutely necessary.

Chapter VIII

The Carbon Monoxide Gasdynamic Laser

8.1 Introduction

All previous sections of this book have dealt exclusively with CO_2–N_2–H_2O or CO_2–N_2–He gas mixtures, with the lasing transition at 10.6 μm. These are the mixtures employed to date in all large scale gasdynamic lasers. However, these are by no means the only possibilities. For example, N_2O has a vibrational energy level structure analogous to CO_2 and possibly could be used as the lasing molecule in N_2O–N_2–H_2O or He mixtures, producing radiation at 10.8 μm. However, the "resonant" or pumping V–V transition between N_2 and N_2O is 107 cm^{-1} compared to 18 cm^{-1} between N_2 and CO_2; thus, N_2O gasdynamic lasers should be far less efficient than CO_2 GDLs. However, of more interest is the use of diatomic molecules as the lasing species in gasdynamic lasers. Examples are CO, HCl, and DCl. These molecules are interesting because (1) the laser wavelengths are much shorter than 10.6 μm, with some transitions corresponding to "windows" in the atmosphere, and (2) some diatomic gasdynamic lasers may be more efficient than conventional CO_2 gasdynamic lasers. Moreover, the physical process creating population inversions in diatomic GDLs is inherently different from that of CO_2 GDLs. This chapter discusses such diatomic GDLs and contrasts them with the conventional CO_2 system. Carbon monoxide will be used as the main example, because the pioneering work of McKenzie (1972) has provided extensive experimental and theoretical results for population inversions and laser power extraction in rapidly expanding CO–N_2–Ar mixtures.

8.2 The Physical Process

The molecular kinetics of CO–N_2–Ar gasdynamic lasers rely upon the freezing of vibrational energy in N_2 and CO in a supersonic expansion. Both CO and N_2 have unusually long relaxation times. Furthermore, vibrational energy is pumped from N_2 ($v = 1$) to CO ($v = 1$), similar to the conventional CO_2–N_2 system. However, the similarity stops there, because the vibrational energy is rapidly distributed *upward* to the higher lying levels of CO due to rapid vibration–vibration (V–V) transfer. The anharmonicity of these upper levels promotes the rapid V–V transfers, as discussed by Treanor *et al.* (1968). The net result is a non-Boltzmann distribution of molecules among the upper CO vibrational levels. This distribution may lead to a vibrational population inversion in the usual sense (more particles in an upper vibrational level than a lower level) or more likely it will result in a partial inversion for a given rotation–vibration transition, even though a total vibrational inversion does not exist.

To see this more clearly, consider the V–V energy exchange given by

$$CO(v) + CO(v) \rightleftarrows CO(v+1) + CO(v-1) + KE \tag{8.1}$$

Here, two CO molecules in the vth vibrational level collide, with the result that one molecule is "pumped up" to the $v + 1$ level while the other drops down to the $v - 1$ level. If the molecules were harmonic oscillators, the vibrational energy levels would be equally spaced, and there would be no change in the kinetic energy of the colliding molecules. However, as illustrated in Fig. 8.1, the vibrational energy levels of CO are in actuality

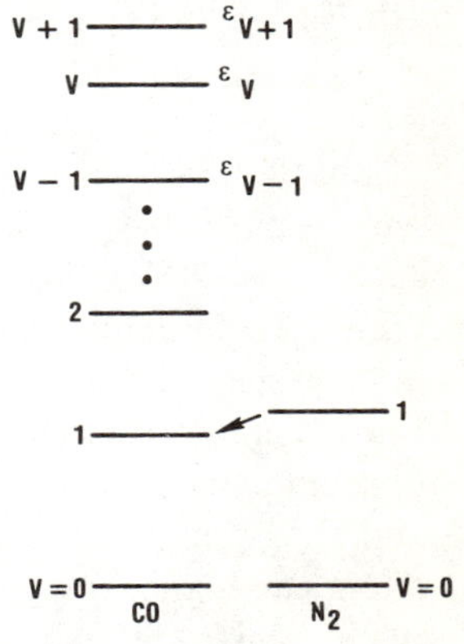

FIG. 8.1 Schematic of vibrational energy levels for CO and N_2.

anharmonic, with continually decreasing spacing as v increases. As a result, the collision process illustrated by the forward reaction (left to right) in Eq. (8.1) yields a small amount of kinetic energy due simply to the unequally spaced anharmonic levels. More specifically, referring to Fig. 8.1,

$$\mathrm{KE} = 2\epsilon_v - \epsilon_{v+1} - \epsilon_{v-1} \tag{8.2}$$

Assuming a Morse internuclear potential, the vibrational energy levels of an anharmonic oscillator are given by McKenzie (1972):

$$\epsilon_v = h\nu v[1 - \epsilon_j(v+1)] \tag{8.3}$$

where ϵ_j is a small anharmonic coefficient, v is the vibrational quantum number, and ν is the fundamental frequency. Substituting Eq. (8.3) into Eq. (8.2),

$$\mathrm{KE} = 2h\nu\epsilon_j \tag{8.4}$$

Thus, the forward reaction of Eq. (8.1) yields a small positive kinetic energy in the amount of $2h\nu\epsilon_j$ per transition. (If the molecules were harmonic oscillators, then $\epsilon_j = 0$, and hence KE = 0.) On the other hand, the reverse reaction (from right to left) in Eq. (8.1) requires a relative kinetic energy of at least $2h\nu\epsilon_j$ to be supplied by the colliding particles. If the temperature of the gas is low enough, the average kinetic energy of the molecules will not be sufficient to allow the reverse reaction. Thus, at low temperatures, *the forward reaction will be favored*, with the net result that molecules are pumped to the higher lying vibrational levels. In turn, this V–V process for anharmonic oscillators will result in an "overpopulation" of the upper levels; i.e., a non-Boltzmann distribution will occur. For this case, Treanor *et al.* (1968) give the population distribution as

$$N_v = N_{v=0} \exp[(\alpha v - \epsilon_v)/kT] \tag{8.5}$$

where α is an anharmonic parameter. Equation (8.5) should be compared with Eq. (3.2) for a harmonic oscillator,

$$N_v = N_{v=0} \exp(-\epsilon_v/kT) \tag{8.6}$$

Equation (8.5) is sometimes labeled as the "Treanor distribution." It assumes only V–V transitions; T–V processes are neglected. Depending on the value of T, the Treanor distribution predicts an overpopulation of the higher lying anharmonic levels sufficient to produce a population inversion above a certain value of v. This is why diatomic molecules have promise in gasdynamic lasers; in a nonequilibrium nozzle expansion, due to the anharmonicity of the molecules, the frozen vibrational energy within CO [and that pumped into CO from N_2 (see Fig. 8.1)] will be redistributed among the higher lying levels with the possibility of creating a population inversion. However, this process will be somewhat compromised by the inclusion of T–V transitions, which will decrease the population of the higher lying levels; indeed, the importance of such T–V deactivation increases as v increases. This tends to limit the application of the Treanor distribution to low values of v, say below $v = 8$ for practical cases.

To make accurate predictions of the anharmonic oscillator population distribution for all important values of v, a master rate equation, similar to Eq. (3.24), must be solved for each level. That is,

$$\begin{aligned} dN_v/dt = {} & (\text{T–V transfers per second from } v+1 \text{ to } v) \\ & + (\text{T–V transfers per second from } v-1 \text{ to } v) \\ & - (\text{T–V transfers per sscond from } v \text{ to } v+1) \\ & - (\text{T–V transfers per second from } v \text{ to } v-1) \\ & + (\text{V–V transfers per second from } v+1 \text{ to } v) \\ & + (\text{V–V transfers per second from } v-1 \text{ to } v) \\ & - (\text{V–V transfers per second from } v \text{ to } v+1) \\ & - (\text{V–V transfers per second from } v \text{ to } v-1) \end{aligned} \tag{8.7}$$

Note that Eq. (8.7) does not include multiple quantum jumps, which are assumed to have a low probability. The V–V transitions affecting the population of the v level are Eq. (8.1) and its counterparts

$$\mathrm{CO}(v+1) + \mathrm{CO}(v+1) \rightleftarrows \mathrm{CO}(v+2) + \mathrm{CO}(v) + \mathrm{KE} \tag{8.8}$$

$$\mathrm{CO}(v-1) + \mathrm{CO}(v-1) \rightleftarrows \mathrm{CO}(v) + \mathrm{CO}(v-2) + \mathrm{KE} \tag{8.9}$$

The precisely resonant transitions such as

$$\mathrm{CO}(v) + \mathrm{CO}(v+1) \rightleftarrows \mathrm{CO}(v+1) + \mathrm{CO}(v)$$

do not have a net effect on N_v and are not included. Using the nomenclature developed in Chapter III, Eq. (8.7) can be written as

$$\begin{aligned} dN_v/dt = {} & \sum_J Z_{\mathrm{C}J}\Big[\overset{v+1,v}{P}(\mathrm{C},J)\,n_{v+1} + \overset{v-1,v}{P}(\mathrm{C},J)\,n_{v-1} \\ & - \overset{v,v+1}{P}(\mathrm{C},J)\,n_v - \overset{v,v-1}{P}(\mathrm{C},J)\,n_v\Big] \\ & + (Z_{\mathrm{CC}}/N_{\mathrm{CO}})\Big[Q(\overset{v+1,v}{\mathrm{C}}, \underset{v+1,v+2}{\mathrm{C}})(n_{v+1})^2 - Q(\overset{v,v+1}{\mathrm{C}}, \underset{v+2,v+1}{\mathrm{C}})\,n_v n_{v+2} \\ & + Q(\overset{v-1,v}{\mathrm{C}}, \underset{v-1,v-2}{\mathrm{C}})(n_{v-1})^2 - Q(\overset{v,v-1}{\mathrm{C}}, \underset{v-2,v-1}{\mathrm{C}})(n_v)(n_{v-2}) \\ & - 2Q(\overset{v,v+1}{\mathrm{C}}, \underset{v,v-1}{\mathrm{C}})(n_v)^2 + 2Q(\overset{v+1,v}{\mathrm{C}}, \underset{v-1,v}{\mathrm{C}})(n_{v-1})(n_{v+1})\Big] \end{aligned} \tag{8.10}$$

where Z_{CJ} is the collision frequency of one CO molecule with molecules of chemical species J, P and Q represent the T–V and V–V transition probabilities respectively (see Chapter III), n_v is the population of the vth level of CO, and N_{CO} is the total number of CO molecules. In Chapter III values for the transition probabilities for a harmonic oscillator are given and used; unfortunately, values for the P's and Q's in Eq. (8.10) for an anharmonic oscillator are not so easily obtained. Some values are discussed by McKenzie (1972), but to date a substantial uncertainty exists, particularly in the V–V transition probabilities. For this reason, no values will be given here; the reader is urged to consult the modern literature for the most recent information.

The simultaneous solution of the system of rate equations given by Eq. (8.10) for all v levels of interest yields the anharmonic oscillator population distribution, accounting for both T–V and V–V transitions. An example of such a solution is given by the solid curve in Fig. 8.2, which also compares results obtained from the Treanor distribution [Eq. (8.5)] and from the harmonic oscillator approximation. These results have been calculated by McKenzie (1972) at an area ratio of $A/A^* = 200$ in a two-dimensional supersonic nozzle expansion of pure CO. Note that the Treanor distribution

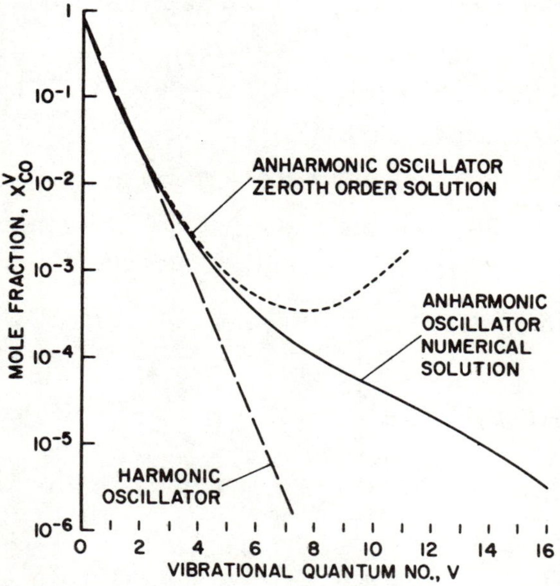

FIG. 8.2 Population distributions at $A/A^* = 200$ for harmonic and anharmonic CO expanding in a two-dimensional supersonic nozzle with a 15° divergence half-angle and a 1.27 mm throat height. $p_0 = 100$ atm; $T_0 = 2000$°K. (After McKenzie, 1972.)

(which accounts for V–V transfers only) predicts a population inversion above $v = 8$, whereas the more accurate solution from Eq. (8.10) (which accounts for both V–V and T–V transitions) shows a considerable overpopulation in comparison to the harmonic oscillator, but no population inversion. Also note that the Treanor distribution is a good approximation at low values of v.

In previous chapters dealing with CO_2–N_2–H_2O or He mixtures and utilizing the harmonic oscillator approximation, vibrational temperatures were defined and were found to be useful quantities. The different vibrational modes of CO_2 were assumed to be in local equilibrium within themselves but not with each other, with different vibrational temperatures for each mode. That is, each mode was assumed to have a local Boltzmann distribution commensurate with its vibrational temperature. In contrast, the anharmonic oscillator population distributions discussed in the present chapter are non-Boltzmann and do not lend themselves to a meaningful single vibrational temperature as defined in previous chapters. Of course, it is possible to define a vibrational temperature for each energy level as

$$N_v = N_0 \exp(-\epsilon_v/kT_v) \tag{8.11}$$

where T_v is different for each value of v. However, because T_{vib} is a function of v, it is not a convenient analytical quantity as in our previous work with CO_2. Nevertheless, it is interesting to note that if a vibrational temperature T_v for anharmonic CO is defined between the $v = 1$ and $v = 0$ levels,

$$N_1 = N_0 \exp(-\epsilon_1/kT_v) \tag{8.12}$$

then in a supersonic nozzle expansion of a CO–N_2 mixture starting from a reservoir temperature T_0, the vibrational temperature can actually climb higher than T_0. This is a ramification of nearly equilibrated V–V exchange between two different species (such as CO and N_2) and is discussed by Treanor *et al.* (1968). It is also pointed out by Teare *et al.* (1970) and is sometimes referred to as the "Teare effect." Such results for a nozzle expansion of CO–N_2 mixtures are calculated by McKenzie and are shown in Fig. 8.3. Here, the vibrational temperature T_v defined by Eq. (8.12) is divided by the reservoir temperature T_0 and is plotted as a function of area ratio (hence distance) through the nozzle for mixtures with different CO contents. The corresponding vibrational temperatures for N_2 are also shown as the dashed curves. Note that T_v(CO) is always larger than $T_v(N_2)$ and is larger than T_0 for some mixtures.

Even though the results in Fig. 8.3 are calculated for anharmonic CO–N_2 mixtures, the "Teare effect" does not depend on anharmonicity; as stated above, it reflects local V–V equilibrium between $v = 1$ levels of CO and N_2. In fact, a simple algebraic relation between T_v(CO) and $T_v(N_2)$

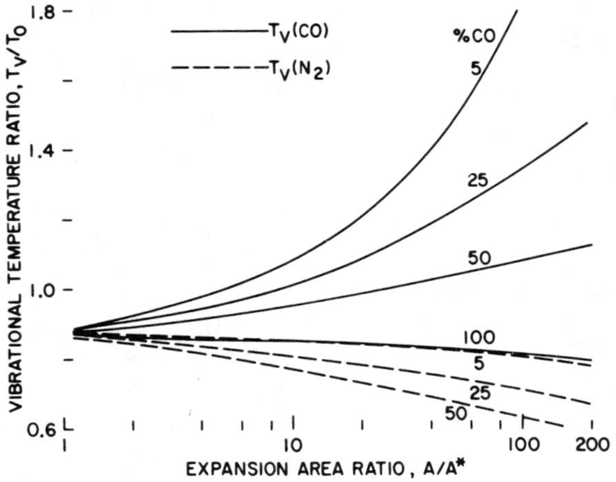

FIG. 8.3 Vibrational temperatures normalized by the reservoir temperature in expansions of anharmonic CO–N_2 mixtures. Nozzle conditions are the same as for Fig. 8.2. (After McKenzie, 1972.)

can be obtained for local V–V equilibrium as

$$T_v(\mathrm{CO}) = \theta_{\mathrm{CO}}/\{[\theta_{\mathrm{N}_2}/T_v(\mathrm{N}_2)] - [(\theta_{\mathrm{N}_2} - \theta_{\mathrm{CO}})/T]\} \tag{8.13}$$

This equation is derived in detail as Eq. (C.8) in Appendix C. Because $\theta_{\mathrm{CO}} < \theta_{\mathrm{N}_2}$, Eq. (8.13) shows that if T is sufficiently small, $T_v(\mathrm{CO}) > T_v(\mathrm{N}_2)$. This is one of the effects shown in Fig. 8.3.

[It should be noted that the Teare effect also influences the CO_2–N_2 process discussed in previous chapters. In reality, it is not precise to assume that $T_{\mathrm{vib\,II}}$ is common to both N_2 and the ν_3 mode of CO_2, as assumed in the simplified kinetic model discussed in Chapter IV. Actually, the vibrational temperature of the ν_3 mode of CO_2 will be slightly less than that for N_2 during the nozzle expansion. However, because $(\theta_{\mathrm{CO}_2(\nu_3)} - \theta_{\mathrm{N}_2})$ is very small, the differences between the two vibrational temperatures will be small, and the assumption of a common $T_{\mathrm{vib\,II}}$ for $CO_2(\nu_3)$ and N_2 during the nozzle expansion is reasonable. This is also clear from the numerical results of Munjee (1972).]

Returning to Fig. 8.2, McKenzie's (1972) calculations show a considerable overpopulation of the higher lying vibrational levels of CO but no population inversion. How, then, can a CO gasdynamic laser produce gain if no inversion exists between the vibrational levels? The answer is found in the fact that the laser transitions are vibration–*rotation* transitions, as discussed in Chapter III, and the rotational population distribution must

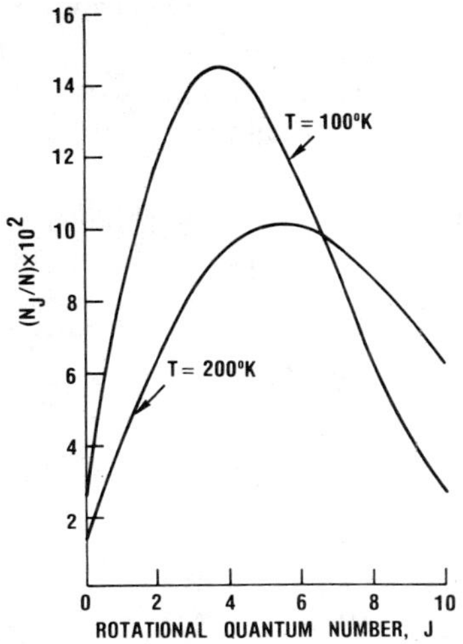

FIG. 8.4

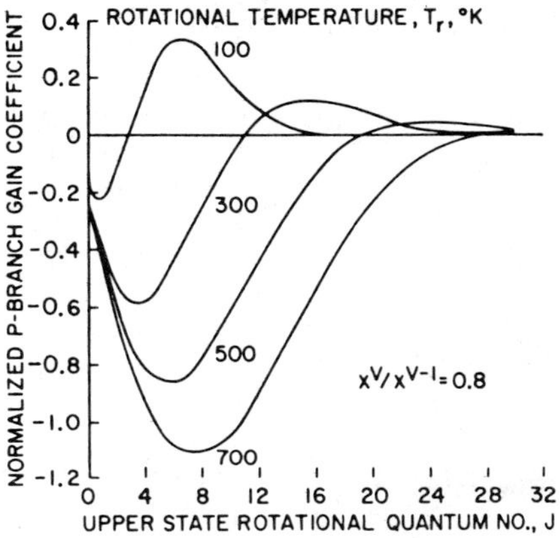

FIG. 8.5

FIG. 8.4 Rotational equilibrium population distribution for two different temperatures.

FIG. 8.5 Normalized P-branch gain coefficients for Doppler-broadened vibration–rotation transitions. Partial inversion case. (After McKenzie, 1972.)

be taken into account. For example, Fig. 8.4 illustrates the equilibrium distribution of particles over the rotational energy levels designated by the quantum number J.

$$N_J/N = (2J + 1)\exp(-\epsilon_J/kT)/Q_{\text{rot}}$$

$$N_J/N = (2J + 1)\left\{\exp\left[\frac{-h^2}{8\pi^2 IkT} J(J + 1)\right]\right\} \Big/ \left(\frac{8\pi^2 IkT}{h^2}\right) \tag{8.14}$$

From Fig. 8.4, or from Eq. (8.14), the ratio $N_{J=8}/N_{J=9} = 1.486$ at $T = 100°\text{K}$. Thus, for a P-branch transition from a vibration–rotation level $(v, J = 8)$ to $(v - 1, J = 9)$, a population inversion may still exist on the strength that $N_J/N_{J+1} > 1$, even though $N_v/N_{v-1} < 1$. Such an inversion is termed a *partial inversion,* in contrast to a total inversion where $N_v/N_{v-1} > 1$. Hence we see that the vibrational population distribution shown as the solid curve in Fig. 8.2, even though it does not indicate a total inversion, does not preclude a partial inversion. Partial inversions are enhanced by low static temperatures because the rotational distribution becomes more peaked at lower temperatures, as shown in Fig. 8.4. In a typical CO gasdynamic laser, the laser gain is derived mainly from a partial inversion, and hence it is necessary to have a low static temperature (generally 100°K or less) in the laser cavity. Gasdynamically, this requires a supersonic nozzle with a large exit-to-throat area ratio.

The influence of partial inversions as calculated by McKenzie (1972) is shown in Fig. 8.5. Here, the P-branch small-signal gain coefficient for CO is plotted versus J for several static temperatures. The ratio $N_v/N_{v-1} = 0.8$; there is no inversion between the vibrational levels; i.e., there is no total inversion. However, there is a partial inversion resulting in laser gain, particularly at lower temperatures.

8.3 Results

McKenzie (1972) has carried out an extensive theoretical and experimental investigation of the CO gasdynamic laser. His results are summarized below.

Theoretical gain calculations are given in Figs. 8.6 and 8.7. Figure 8.6 shows the influence of adding N_2 to CO. The pure CO case (100% CO) in Fig. 8.6 shows a small value of gain; on the other hand, a 25% CO–75% N_2 mixture shows a considerable increase in gain. This is due to the pumping of vibrational energy from frozen N_2 to the $v = 1$ level of CO, and then

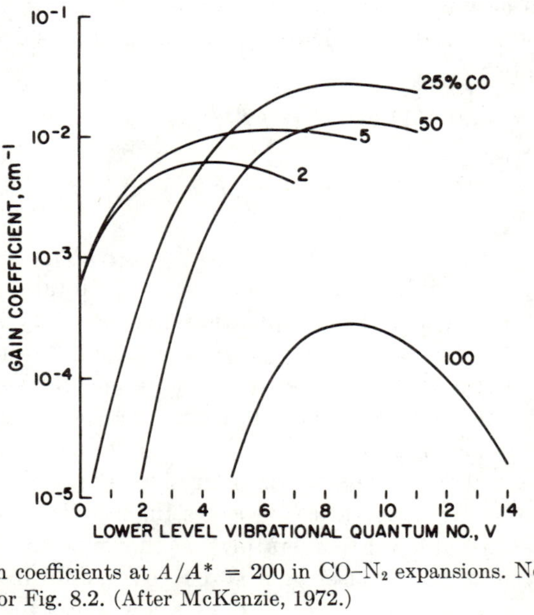

FIG. 8.6 Gain coefficients at $A/A^* = 200$ in CO–N_2 expansions. Nozzle conditions are the same as for Fig. 8.2. (After McKenzie, 1972.)

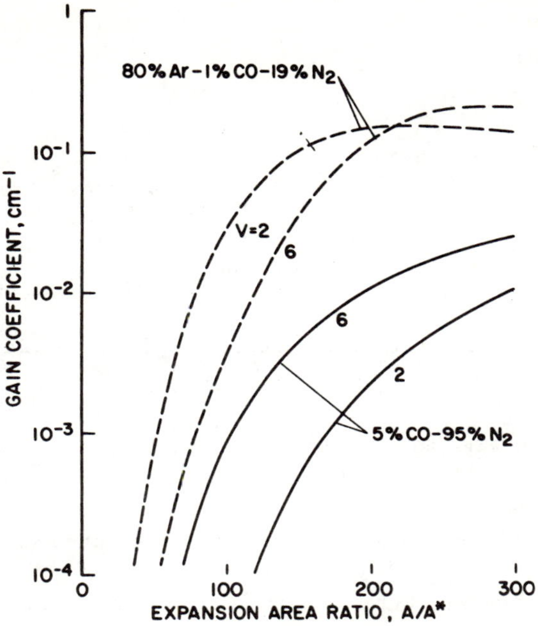

FIG. 8.7 The effect of Ar dilution on CO gain coefficients in N_2–CO–Ar expansions. V is the upper-level vibrational quantum number. Nozzle conditions are the same as for Fig. 8.2. (After McKenzie, 1972.)

up the CO vibrational energy ladder via the anharmonic effect discussed in the previous section. The effect of decreased static temperature, hence increased partial inversions, is shown indirectly in Fig. 8.7. If Ar is mixed with the CO–N_2 gas, the static temperature at any given area ratio in the nozzle will be reduced. This is strictly a thermodynamic effect. Ar is a monatomic gas with a larger isentropic exponent than CO–N_2; hence, the thermodynamics of the supersonic nozzle expansion results in lower values of T. Consequently, the gain coefficient is greatly enhanced by adding Ar to the CO gasdynamic laser. This is clearly seen in Fig. 8.7, which compares a CO–N_2–Ar mixture (dashed curves) with a CO–N_2 mixture (solid curves).

McKenzie (1972) has carried out a series of experiments using a shock tunnel equipped with an axisymmetric 10° half-angle conical nozzle. Mirror ports with their optical axis normal to the flow direction were placed at various downstream locations in the nozzle. Using circular mirrors in these ports, laser power was extracted at these locations. Laser oscillation occurred simultaneously over a number of vibration–rotation transitions with wavelengths ranging from 4.8 to 5.3 μm. The measured variations of

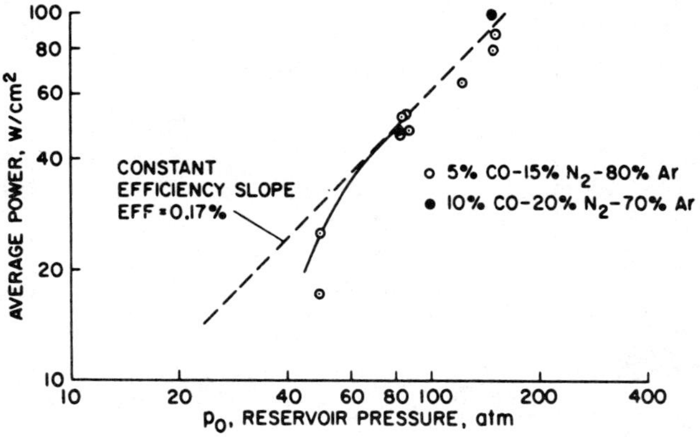

FIG. 8.8 Effect of reservoir pressure on laser energy flux. Test conditions were T_0 = 2100°K, A/A^* = 577, h^* = 1.27 cm. (After McKenzie, 1972.)

the net laser power with reservoir pressure and temperature are shown in Figs. 8.8 and 8.9, respectively, for CO–N_2–Ar mixtures. In each case, the results are obtained at an area ratio of 577. In addition, McKenzie (1972) has defined a laser efficiency as the measured laser power output divided by the fraction of flow total enthalpy convected through the laser beam in-

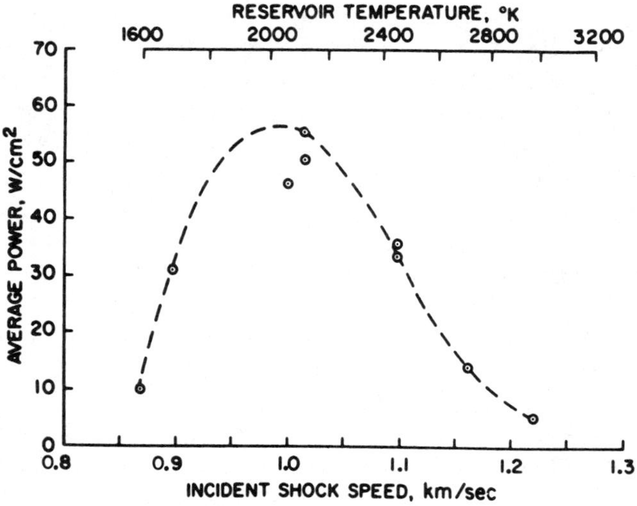

FIG. 8.9 Effect of reservoir temperature on laser energy flux. Test conditions are 5% CO, 15% N_2, 80% Ar, p_0 = 90 atm, A/A^* = 577, h^* = 1.27 cm. (After McKenzie, 1972.)

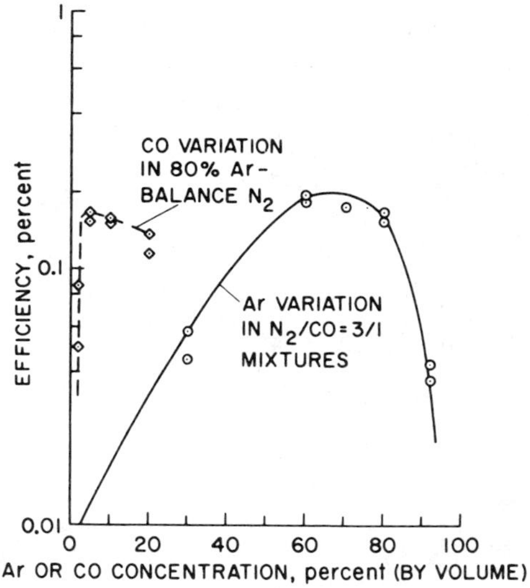

FIG. 8.10 Effect of gas composition on laser efficiency. Test conditions are $p_0 = 85$ atm, $T_0 = 2100°K$, $A/A^* = 577$, $h^* = 1.27$ cm. (After McKenzie, 1972.)

ternally in the cavity. Results for this efficiency as a function of Ar content are shown in Fig. 8.10. This figure demonstrates two important points:

(1) The values of efficiency, though low on the basis of absolute magnitude, are higher than the same figure of merit for conventional CO_2–N_2 GDLs. This is one reason for interest in CO gasdynamic lasers.

(2) The experimental measurements confirm the previous theoretical predictions that Ar is very beneficial to the laser process by reducing the static temperature, hence improving the partial inversions. In fact, the left-hand curve in Fig. 8.10 indicates that the addition of Ar to CO is much more important than the addition of N_2.

8.4 Disadvantage

The CO gasdynamic laser suffers from one practical disadvantage—the requirement for high Mach number flows. The population inversions in CO are enhanced by very low translational temperatures of the gas, on the order of 60°K. In order to achieve such a low temperature, the flow must be expanded in supersonic nozzles with area ratios (exit-to-throat area) on the order of 500—a factor of 10 larger than conventional GDLs. To an aerodynamicist, this implies high Mach number flows with large total pressure losses. Since many practical applications of GDLs involve exhausting the gas to the atmosphere, then either extremely high reservoir pressures are required or a dramatic breakthrough in supersonic diffuser technology is necessary. This amounts to a serious limitation on the practical use of such lasers. However, as described above, there are some compensating advantages, and interest in diatomic gasdynamic lasers should continue to grow in the future.

Chapter IX

Downstream Mixing Gasdynamic Lasers

9.1 Introduction

How do we squeeze the most out of the gasdynamic laser concept? The answer to this question may rest in some recent work on downstream mixing GDLs, which represents the *frontier* of gasdynamic laser research today.

Consider a conventional CO_2–N_2–H_2O or He GDL as discussed in previous chapters and as shown schematically in Fig. 9.1a. Recall that the primary reservoir of energy for laser extraction is in the *vibrationally excited* N_2, even though the laser emission itself occurs via the CO_2 molecules. Of course, one purpose of the supersonic nozzle expansion is to freeze as much of this vibrational energy as possible. *Pure* N_2 has an extremely long relaxation time; hence it readily freezes in a rapid expansion. However, in a conventional GDL, where both CO_2 and H_2O (or He) are present with N_2 in the nozzle expansion, such molecules act as a *contaminant* to the N_2. As a result, the CO_2–N_2–H_2O or He mixture relaxes faster than pure N_2, giving lower vibrational temperatures and hence lower available laser power. This is shown schematically in Fig. 9.2, where the solid curve represents the N_2 vibrational temperature for a conventional GDL contrasted with the dashed curve for the expansion of pure N_2.

In addition to the above consideration, the reservoir temperature T_0 should be made as high as possible in order to obtain maximum laser

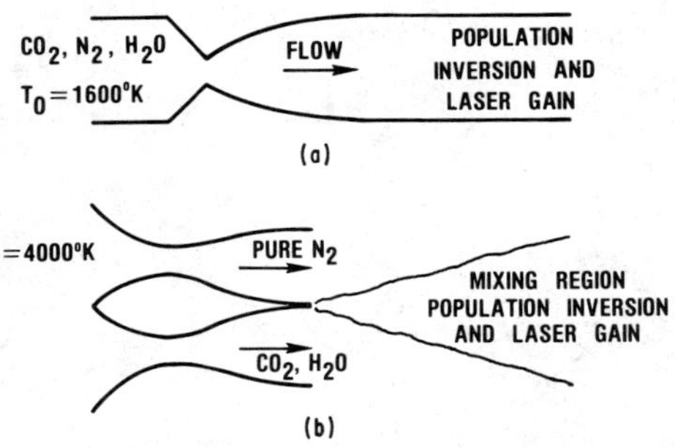

FIG. 9.1 Schematics for conventional and downstream mixing gasdynamic lasers.

power; this is discussed in Chapter VII. The higher the temperature, the more vibrational energy is present in the gas, and subsequently more laser power can be obtained. However, in conventional GDLs, T_0 is limited to values around 2300°K; above this temperature CO_2 begins to chemically dissociate, and laser performance begins to deteriorate. This is in contrast to the dissociation of N_2, which occurs above 4000°K.

In light of the above discussion, there are clearly two major advantages in constructing a gasdynamic laser that expands *pure* N_2 through a supersonic nozzle and then mixes CO_2 and H_2O or He *downstream* of the nozzle exit, namely:

(1) Reservoir temperatures of N_2 can exceed 4000°K, and
(2) More efficient freezing of the N_2 vibrational energy is obtained.

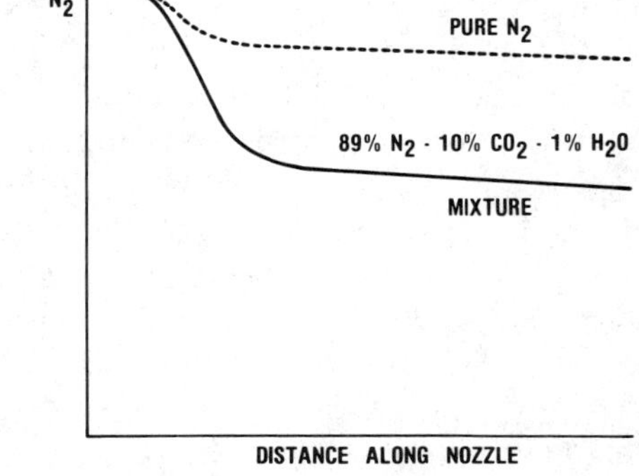

FIG. 9.2 Comparison of N_2 vibrational temperatures for expansions of pure N_2 and for a standard CO_2–N_2–H_2O mixture.

FIG. 9.3 Schematic of a simple downstream mixing gasdynamic laser.

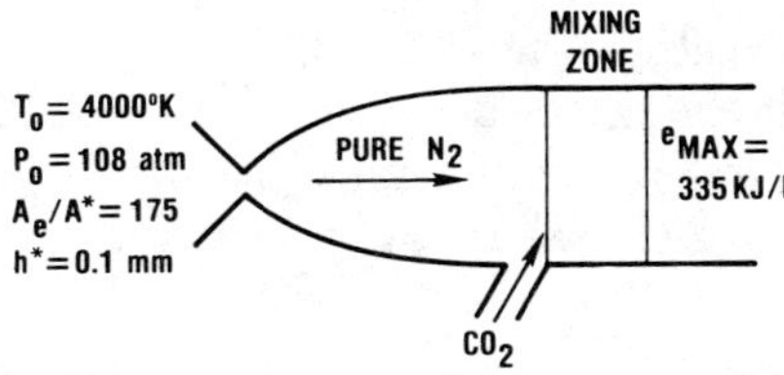

Such a device is called a *downstream mixing gasdynamic laser*, and it is shown schematically in Fig. 9.1b. Here two parallel mixing streams are shown, one with pure vibrationally excited N_2 and the other with cold CO_2 and H_2O or He. Downstream of the nozzle exits, the two streams mix, and the vibrationally excited N_2 molecules collide with and transfer energy to the CO_2. Under suitable conditions, substantial gain and power extraction can be obtained.

To see this more clearly, consider the almost normal injection of CO_2 into a supersonic stream of pure N_2 as shown schematically in Fig. 9.3. If the ideal situation of instantaneous mixing is assumed, then, for the conditions shown in Fig. 9.3, a nonequilibrium calculation using the method of Glowacki and Anderson (1971) indicates a maximum available power of over 300 kJ/lb_m. This is an order of magnitude improvement over the existing second-generation GDLs discussed in Chapter VII. In fact, this result is compared with other laser concepts in Fig. 9.4. Here, typical specific energies of conventional first- and second-generation GDLs,

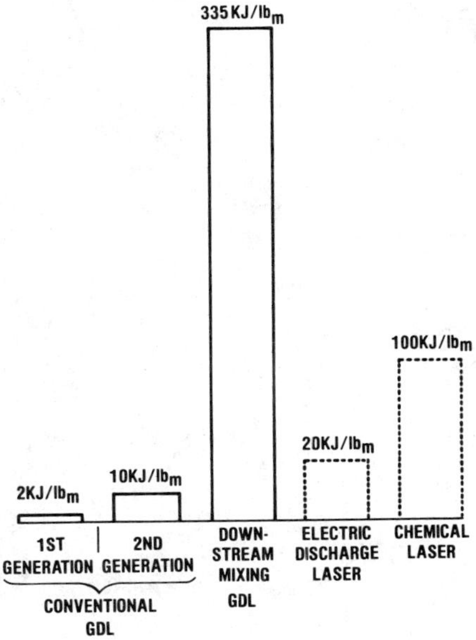

FIG. 9.4 Comparison of specific power for the downstream mixing gasdynamic laser with other laser types.

electric discharge lasers, and chemical lasers are contrasted with the downstream mixing GDL. The comparison shown in Fig. 9.4 is not quite fair, however, because the 335 kJ/lb_m shown for the downstream mixing GDL is a highly idealized value. However, Fig. 9.4 clearly dramatizes why there is current interest in such devices.

9.2 Problems

There are obvious practical problems associated with downstream mixing GDLs. For example, mixing does not occur instantaneously; hence throughout the finite mixing region of a real flow, vibrational deactivation will constantly decrease the available power. Some numerical results for the turbulent parallel mixing of streams of N_2 and CO_2 are shown in Fig. 9.5. Here, the mass fraction profiles of N_2 across the two streams is shown at various axial locations. These results are obtained from unpublished calculations by the author's laser research group at the University of Maryland, where studies of the downstream mixing GDLs are being made by solving the complete Navier–Stokes equations using a time-dependent finite-difference technique analogous to that described in Chapter IV. The profiles shown in Fig. 9.5 clearly indicate the finite extent of the mixing zone. The question is: Does enough deactivation occur within this finite zone to negate the whole concept? Work is being done to answer this question, as described in Section 9.3.

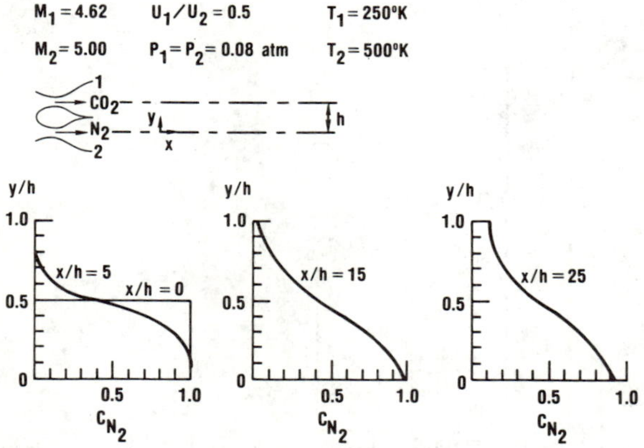

FIG. 9.5 N_2 mass fraction profiles for turbulent mixing at various axial locations along the flow for a downstream mixing gasdynamic laser.

There are other problems with downstream mixing GDLs. For example, can the nozzles be made of materials that can withstand such high temperatures in the small nozzle throats? How can we produce N_2 at 4000°K on a continued, practical basis? Also, recall that high Mach number nozzles are required to insure that the gas translational temperature (hence the lower laser level population) in the cavity will be low. Hence can diffusers be developed that will allow exhausting the flow to the atmosphere? Can the flows be mixed without inducing strong shock waves or major turbulence in the laser cavity that degrade beam quality?

9.3 Results

The advantage of high power output obtained in a downstream mixing GDL encourages work on this concept, even in the face of the above problems. Some early experimental work has been performed by Bronfin *et al.* (1970) using arc-heated N_2 with CO_2–He injected vertically into the supersonic flow in the cavity. Their results were the first to demonstrate the potential of the downstream mixing concept. However, this work was not pursued, presumably due to concern about shock waves, hence poor beam quality, in the cavity. More recently, downstream mixing GDL experiments using *tangential* mixing in a shock tube have been reported by Milewski *et al.* (1972). Chroshko *et al.* (1972, 1973) report some interesting results obtained by injecting cold CO_2 and He slightly downstream of the sonic region of an expansion of pure N_2. Also, Howgate *et al.* (1972) report

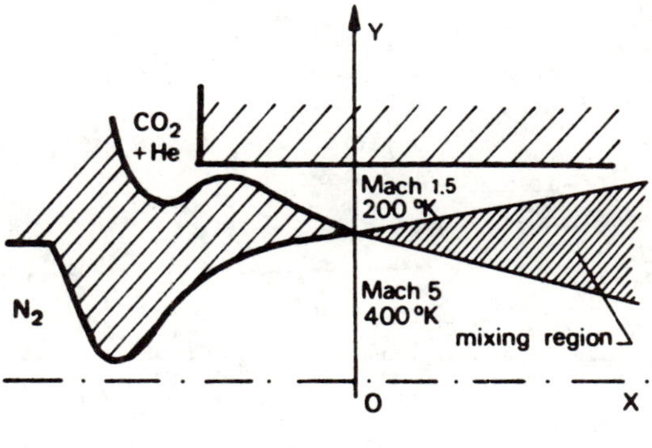

FIG. 9.6 Schematic showing supersonic mixing downstream of the nozzle exit. (After Taran *et al.*, 1973.)

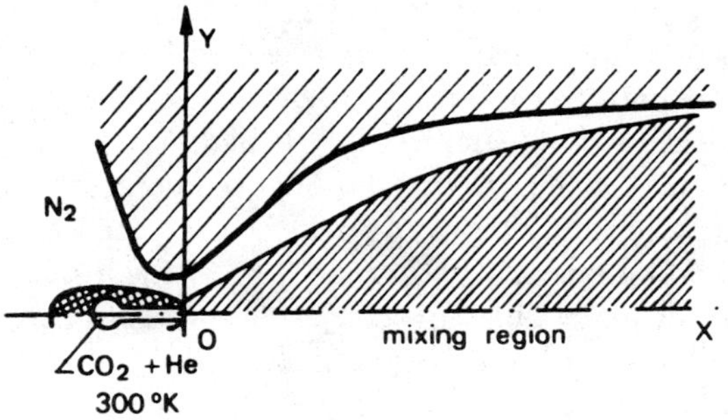

FIG. 9.7 Schematic showing mixing in the throat region. (After Taran *et al.*, 1973.)

some similar measurements with CO_2 injected both at the nozzle exit and upstream of the throat.

However, the most complete investigations by far have been conducted by the team of Borghi and Charpenel (1972), who have performed detailed vibrational nonequilibrium flow field calculations of tangential downstream mixing using a finite-difference solution of the turbulent boundary layer equations, and by Taran *et al.* (1973), who report a systematic series of arc-tunnel experiments complementing the theoretical predictions. Some of the results of Taran *et al.* (1973) are shown in Figs. 9.6–9.11. They examined mixing downstream of the nozzle exit (Fig. 9.6) as well as mixing in the throat region (Fig. 9.7). Theoretical results for gain profiles are shown in Fig. 9.8 for mixing downstream of the exit. For this case the cal-

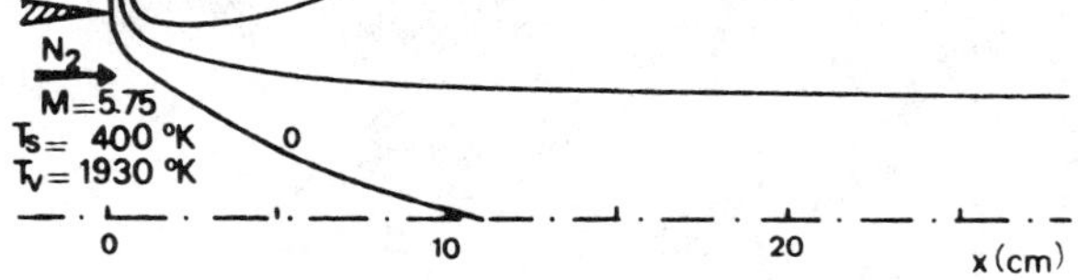

FIG. 9.8 Calculated small-signal gain contours for mixing downstream of the nozzle exit. The upper flow is originally 10% CO_2, 90% He. Gain is calculated on the P(30) line. (After Taran *et al.*, 1973.)

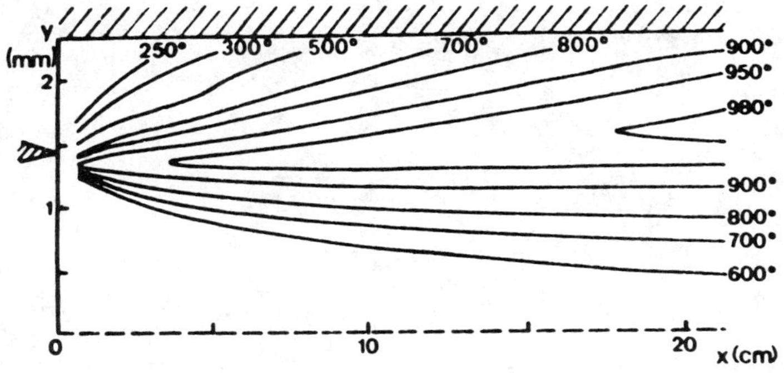

FIG. 9.9 Calculated static temperature contours for mixing downstream of the nozzle exit. (After Taran *et al.*, 1973.)

culated gain was disappointingly low; indeed, the values shown in Fig. 9.8 hardly match the small-signal gain achieved in conventional gas-dynamic lasers. The problem is caused by a recovery of a substantial portion of the N_2 stream total temperature in the mixing region, leading to high static temperatures (800 to 1000°K) hence low gains. (Recall from Chapters III and IV that a low static temperature is necessary to keep the lower laser level in CO_2 relatively depopulated.) To see this more clearly, consider Fig. 9.9. Here calculated contours of static temperature illustrate the high temperatures in the mixing region and clearly explain the low gains shown in Fig. 9.8. Taran's (1973) arc tunnel experiments also confirm the low gain in this case. On the other hand, a considerable improvement is

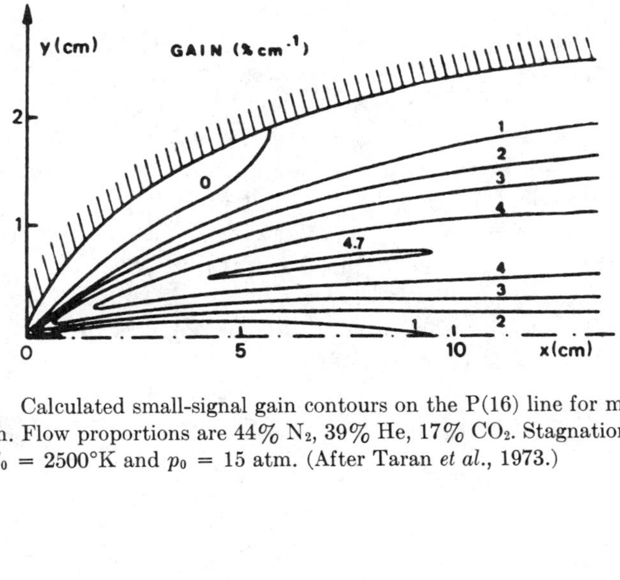

FIG. 9.10 Calculated small-signal gain contours on the P(16) line for mixing in the throat region. Flow proportions are 44% N_2, 39% He, 17% CO_2. Stagnation conditions for N_2 are T_0 = 2500°K and p_0 = 15 atm. (After Taran *et al.*, 1973.)

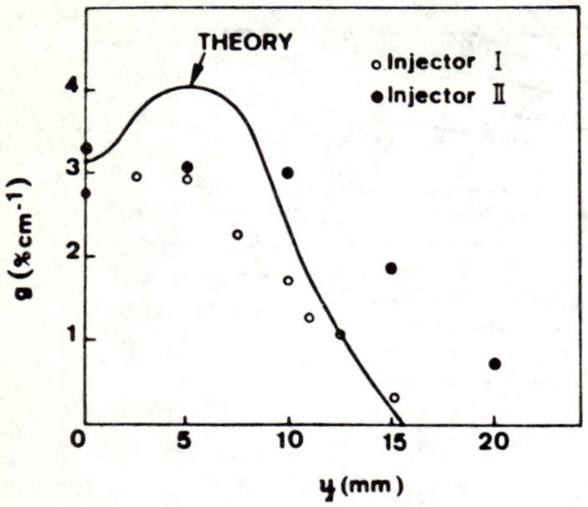

FIG. 9.11 Measured small-signal gain distributions across the flow at 15 cm downstream of the throat. Case for mixing in the throat region. (After Taran *et al.*, 1973.)

obtained with injection in the throat region (Fig. 9.7). For this case calculated results for small-signal gain are shown in Fig. 9.10. An order of magnitude improvement is apparent. The experimental results for gain shown in Fig. 9.11 confirm these calculations. With injection in the throat region, relatively uniform mixing takes place early enough in the expansion that the high static temperatures discussed above are not obtained, thus leading to increased gain.

Injection in the throat region is still a compromise of the ultimate downstream mixing advantage, because collisional deactivation of the vibrationally excited N_2 will be increased downstream of the injection region. That is, the advantage of having a complete expansion of pure N_2, hence the best freezing efficiency, is compromised. Also, if the N_2 reservoir temperature is 4000°K or higher, then the static temperature in the throat region will still be high enough to cause some dissociation of CO_2. That is, the advantage of having the highest possible reservoir temperature is also compromised by injection in the throat region. Therefore, mixing downstream of the nozzle exit is still an attractive concept, as long as efforts are made to maintain a low static temperature in the mixing region. This can be achieved by closer matching of the two stream velocities. Admittedly, this will also tend to decrease the rate of mixing; however, the mixing rate can be increased by other means, such as increasing the level of turbulence in the nozzle boundary layer and in the free stream. These considerations are presently at the frontier of the state-of-the-art, and much research still remains to be accomplished before the full potential of the downstream mixing gasdynamic laser is assessed.

Chapter X

Optical Cavity Considerations for Gasdynamic Lasers

10.1 Introduction

The previous chapters have emphasized the gasdynamic and vibrational kinetic aspects of gasdynamic lasers that bear on the generation of population inversions, small-signal gain, and power extraction. In particular, Chapter IV treats the calculation of power extraction essentially as a case of solving the radiative transfer equation $dI/I = G\,dy$ between mirrors in the cavity, coupled with the nonequilibrium supersonic flow. Such calculations generally provide results on the raw power output available from the cavity. However, the total picture of power extraction is more than that. It is also a matter of considering the *optical* design of the cavity, taking into account the actual path of the light rays (geometric optics), mirror losses (such as absorption), diffraction (physical optics), and the density inhomogeneities of the flowing gas that cause phase distortions in the laser beam. In essence the basic philosophy of optical cavity design is stated by Clark (1972): "Achieve the maximum output power in a beam with minimum divergence, limited only by diffraction." Such considerations are the subject of this chapter.

Emphasis is made that the optical phase distribution across the output beam from a laser cavity should be constant (uniphase) and that the beam divergence angle should be as small as nature allows (limited only by diffraction through the output aperture). For these conditions the laser beam can be focused to a spot of minimum diameter. Any deviation from these conditions will reduce the beam intensity in the far field.

Finally, the purpose of this chapter is not to give a treatise on laser optical cavities; such matters are treated by such authors as Siegman (1971) and Lengyel (1971). Rather, the intent here is to discuss those aspects of laser cavities that are particularly germane to gasdynamic lasers.

10.2 Cavity Types

(a) Amplifiers

The first generation of GDLs has extracted power by using the cavity as an amplifier, such as shown in Fig. 10.1. Here an independent beam from a CO_2 laser (usually a "conventional" electric discharge laser) is fed into the GDL cavity through an input aperture. This CO_2 laser is called the master oscillator (MO). The beam is then reflected back and forth inside the GDL cavity for several passes, being amplified by the laser medium on each pass. On the last pass the beam leaves the cavity either through small holes in the output mirror or through some type of window. At

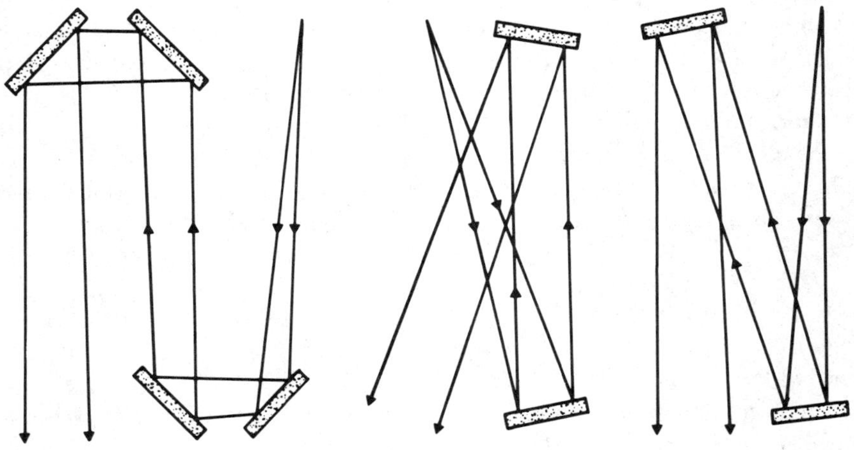

FIG. 10.1 Typical MOPA folding geometries. (After Clark, 1972.)

present extracting the last pass through a solid window is impractical because current window materials cannot tolerate the high heating loads imposed by the high power beam. This leads to the use of aerodynamic windows, to be discussed in Chapter XI. Referring again to Fig. 10.1, the cavity is acting as a power amplifier (PA), and the whole arrangement of oscillator and cavity is called the master oscillator power amplifier (MOPA). The number and arrangement of passes through the cavity depend on the designer's intentions; several possible geometries are shown in Fig. 10.1, which is taken from Clark (1972).

There are three major advantages of the MOPA for extracting power:

(a) The input beam from the master oscillator, assuming it is properly designed, is already in constant phase. Hence if the amplifier medium in the cavity is homogeneous, then the output beam should also be of constant phase.

(b) The power level of the output beam of a MOPA can be readily increased or decreased simply by controlling the input beam from the MO. This adds a certain flexibility to GDL operation.

(c) The timewise (temporal) variation of the output beam can also be controlled in a similar manner.

Referring again to Fig. 10.1, a disadvantage of the MOPA is that most of the power available in the supersonic gas in the cavity is extracted only during the last beam pass; the role of the other passes is simply to build up the intensity so that the last pass reaches saturation intensity. At saturation intensity the beam is extracting energy from the CO_2 molecules just as fast as the N_2 can pump energy into the upper laser level (001) of CO_2. In the meantime during the earlier beam passes that occur upstream of the last, saturating pass, available laser energy in the gas is being lost due to collisional deactivation of the molecules. Hence a MOPA arrangement is in general an *inefficient* way of extracting the available laser energy.

(b) Resonators

A resonator is a self-contained extraction device in which the laser radiation is initially triggered by random spontaneous emission and then rapidly increased by stimulated emission in a direction perpendicular to mirrors on both sides of the cavity. Three types of resonators are shown in Fig. 10.2, taken from Clark (1972). Resonators have the advantage of rapidly building up saturation intensity within the cavity, hence being more efficient in general than the MOPA discussed above. They have the disadvantage of allowing no intensity control, and the optical alignment

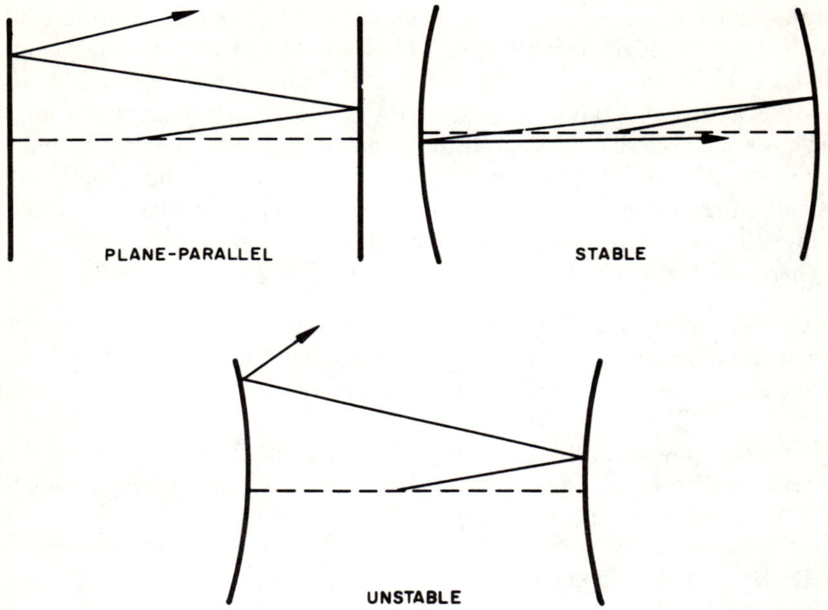

FIG. 10.2 Types of laser resonators. (After Clark, 1972.)

is more difficult than MOPA's. However, their efficient operation, which is related to their ability to extract energy in a short flow length, makes such resonators of extreme interest in GDL design.

There are basically three types of resonators, and they all have been used at one time or another on a GDL. These types are shown in Fig. 10.2. The major distinction between them is that light rays that are slightly off-axis tend to "walk out" of the plane-parallel and unstable resonators but are contained by the stable resonator.

Diffraction plays a very important role in determining what type of intensity pattern exists in the output laser beam that emerges from the output mirror. As stated by Clark (1972), to produce a phase coherent beam, all parts of the laser cavity should share energy through diffraction. In this way the optical phases of all the emitting molecules are locked together through cross-coupling within the cavity, and a laser beam of the lowest order transverse mode will be produced. Some cavities do this job better than others. For example, a number of laser transverse modes can oscillate within a cavity, each producing a different intensity pattern in the output beam. The intensity patterns associated with twelve of these modes are shown in Fig. 10.3, which is taken from Kogelnik and Li (1966). The

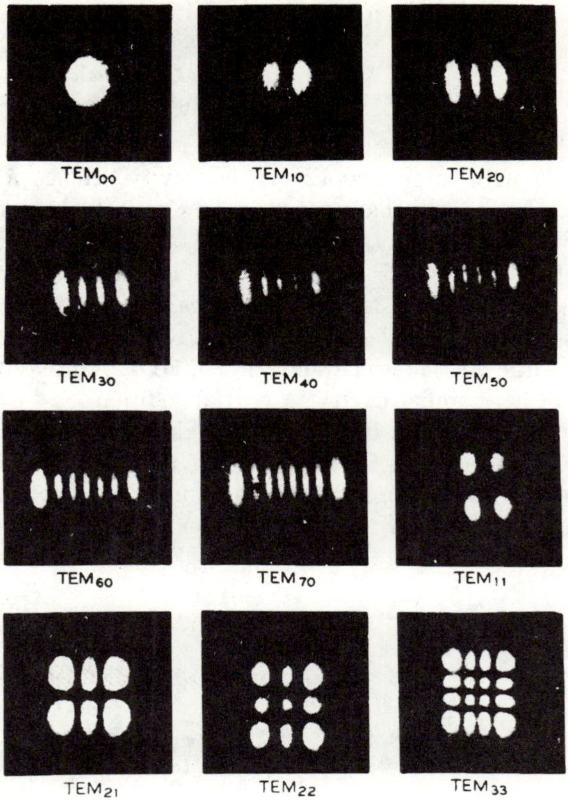

FIG. 10.3 Mode patterns of a gas laser oscillator. (After Kogelnik and Li, 1966.)

best quality laser beam is one where a single mode is operating, with that mode being the *lowest order* TEM_{00} mode. (TEM means transverse electromagnetic mode.) This mode produces the single spot seen in the upper left corner of Fig. 10.3. Unfortunately, it is very difficult to obtain single mode operation; indeed, most GDLs have in the past operated multimode.

What is the problem that causes multimode operation? First, consider a stable resonator and define the Fresnel number N_F as $N_F = r^2/d\lambda$, where r is the mirror radius, d the distance between mirrors, and λ the laser wavelength. Stable resonators with high and low Fresnel numbers are shown in Fig. 10.4. Diffraction effects in the long cavity (the low Fresnel number cavity) are stronger. This can be seen by inspection of Fig. 10.4, where a slightly off-axis ray effectively has a long enough distance between mirrors

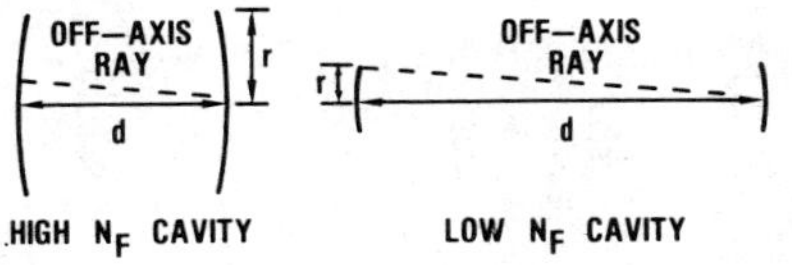

FIG. 10.4 High and low Fresnel number cavities.

to cross-couple with large regions of the cavity. Hence a low Fresnel number cavity has a good chance of operating with the lowest order mode. On the other hand, again looking at Fig. 10.4, the opposite is true of a high Fresnel number cavity. This is also seen in Fig. 10.5, taken from Clark (1972). For a large N_F, the stable resonator can set up several independent modes of operation, with little cross-coupling by diffraction. Unfortunately, to handle the large mass flow characteristic of GDLs, the cavity has to be a fairly high Fresnel number cavity. A partial solution is to use an *unstable* resonator, as shown in Fig. 10.5. Even though N_F may be large, the rays of an unstable resonator spread out within the cavity and provide the desirable strong cross-coupling. Hence, in an unstable resonator, it is more difficult for the higher order transverse modes to oscillate.

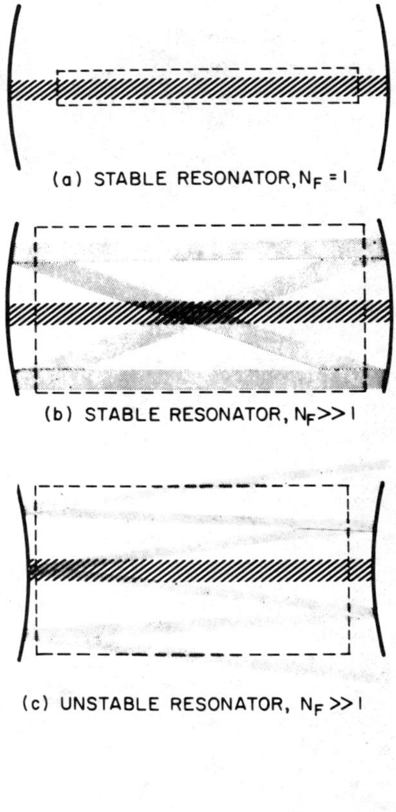

FIG. 10.5 Transverse mode selection for various resonator configurations. (After Clark, 1972.)

10.3 Causes of Beam Distortion in Gasdynamic Lasers

All of the preceeding discussion has assumed that the laser medium (the supersonic flow in the cavity) is homogeneous. If the medium is not homogeneous, then additional sources of phase distortion are present. These additional sources are examined below.

(a) Shock Waves

There are two principal sources of shock waves in the GDL cavity, and these are shown in Fig. 10.6, taken from Simons (1972). The nozzle of a GDL is really a bank of small nozzles in a row—small nozzles to promote vibrational freezing in the expansion. This is shown in the top sketch of Fig. 10.6, which looks down on the top view of a GDL. Here we see the minimum length contour of such nozzles, as well as a diamond shock pattern coming from the nozzle tips. Flow is from left to right, and the laser beam is

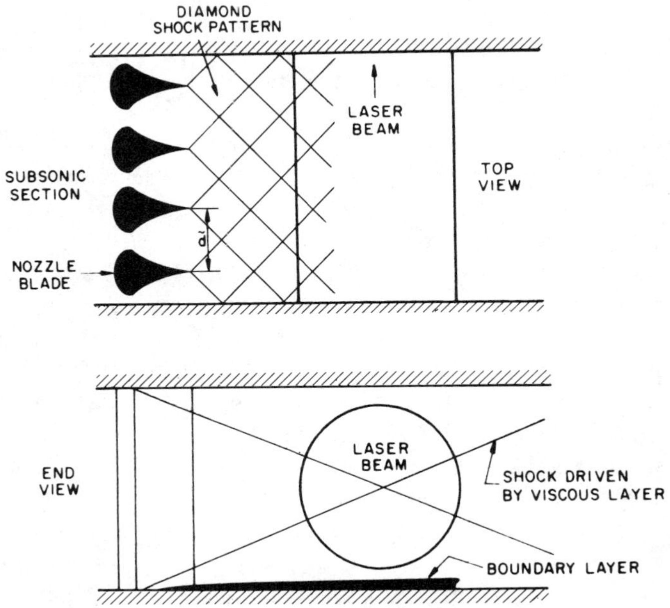

FIG. 10.6 Top and side (end) views of shock patterns in gasdynamic laser cavities. (After Simons, 1972.)

transverse to the flow as shown. The flow at the exit of each nozzle is not exactly parallel; this is due to truncation of the nozzles to obtain structural strength at the tips and to the boundary layer growth along the nozzle walls as well as the wake growth downstream of the tips. Hence a diamond shock pattern is always a characteristic of such multinozzles and was observed long before the advent of gasdynamic lasers (Royle *et al.*, 1947). A detailed survey of these disturbances, as well as other fluid dynamic aspects of gasdynamic lasers, can be found in the recent, excellent survey by Russell (1974).

This diamond shock pattern is generally weak. Moreover, if the laser beam cuts across these shocks in the direction shown in the top of Fig. 10.6, then the optical path will be essentially the same for each ray, and phase distortion will be minimized. Hence the shocks emanating from the nozzle tips are not a major problem.

This is not the case for the shocks that come from the top and bottom walls of the nozzle array. Such shocks are shown in the bottom sketch of Fig. 10.6. Here we are looking at a side view of the GDL, where the nozzle entrance, throat, and exit are shown as the vertical lines. Flow is still from left to right. Consider the expansion in the nozzles. The pressure, density, and temperature drop so rapidly in the nozzle throat region that the boundary layer displacement thickness on the flat top and bottom walls experiences an almost discontinuous increase. This appears as a compression corner to the flow and triggers the two oblique shocks emanating from the top and bottom walls shown in Fig. 10.6. Here the rays of the laser beam are parallel to the plane of the shocks, and the optical length of the rays can vary substantially across the beam, depending on the density of the different regions of the shock pattern. As a result, these top and bottom shocks can cause substantial phase distortion.

There are two solutions to this problem. One is gasdynamic and is discussed by Simons (1972). It involves the simple aspect of contouring the top and bottom walls in the nozzle throat region in such a fashion as to cancel the displacement thickness growth. This is illustrated in Fig. 10.7, taken from Simons (1972). However, precise contouring of the top and bottom walls is a serious fabrication complication for the construction of GDLs. A compromise is discussed by Director (1973), who shows experimentally that the oblique shock waves can be sufficiently mitigated by simply diverging the top and bottom walls by a constant small angle on the order of a degree or so.

The other solution is optical. Hoffman and Jones (1972) have suggested the phase cancellation optical configuration shown in Fig. 10.8. This is characterized by a symmetric beam path arrangement wherein each ray cuts the shock waves an equal number of times and each pass traverses

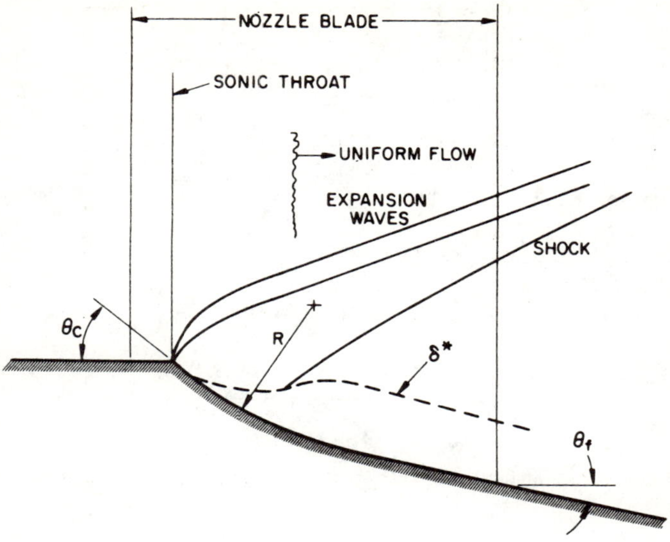

FIG. 10.7 Contour in the top and bottom walls in the throat region of a gasdynamic laser nozzle in order to minimize shock waves. (After Simons, 1972.)

the flow at the same angle. Such an arrangement applies, of course, to the MOPA type of optical cavity design; it is not really applicable to resonators. This phase cancellation idea has led to an order of magnitude improvement in beam quality (Hoffman and Jones, 1972) and is illustrated in Fig. 10.9, obtained from Russell (1974).

As a result of both the above solutions, the serious beam quality problems

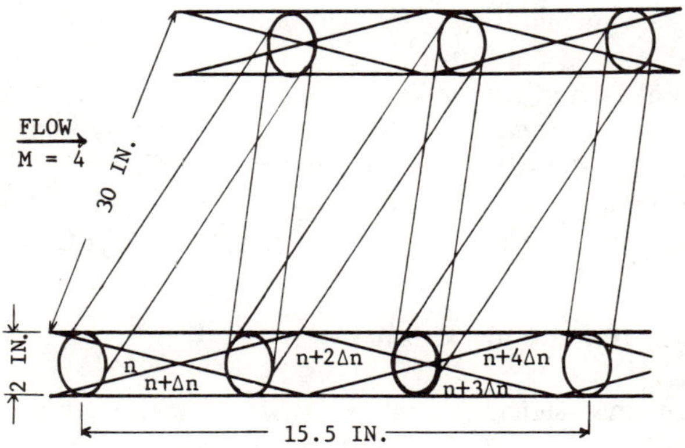

FIG. 10.8 Phase cancellation optical configuration. (After Hoffman and Jones, 1972.)

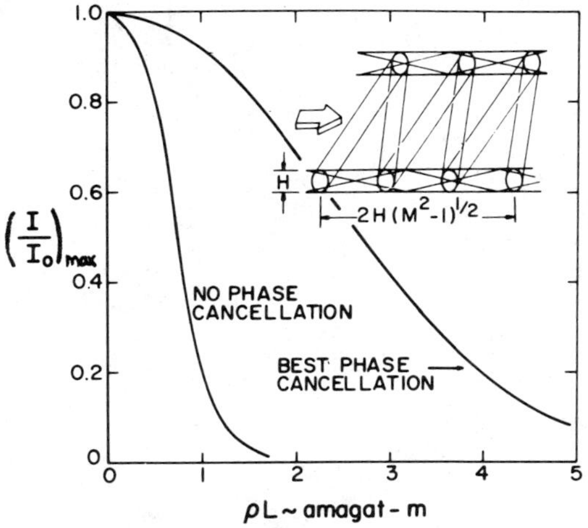

FIG. 10.9 Peak far-field intensity with and without phase cancellation. (After Russell, 1974.)

originally encountered with the cavity shock waves have gradually been minimized. In fact, in a properly designed "clean flow" nozzle and cavity, random turbulence in the flow instead of the shock waves may be the limiting factor on beam quality.

(b) Turbulence

At the present time, there is not much that can be said about turbulence and its quantitative effect on phase distortion. Given the extent and spectrum of the turbulence of the flow in the cavity, the analysis of Sutton (1969) allows a calculation of its effect on the beam in the far field. However, a prediction of the turbulence level generated within the boundary layers and wakes, and that which propagates downstream from the reservoir and subsonic portions of the nozzles, is difficult to obtain. However, we can categorically state that random turbulence will always create a temporal phase change distortion in the beam and that such turbulence can be the fundamental limiting factor in obtaining the best beam quality.

(c) Nonuniform Gain Profiles

Recall that small-signal gain in a GDL varies with distance, as shown in Fig. 5.12, and as sketched in Fig. 10.10 for cases with and without power extraction. Clearly, gain varies through the cavity and across the laser

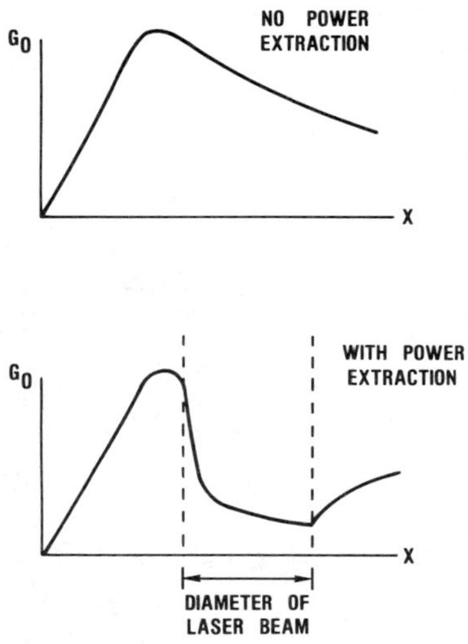

FIG. 10.10

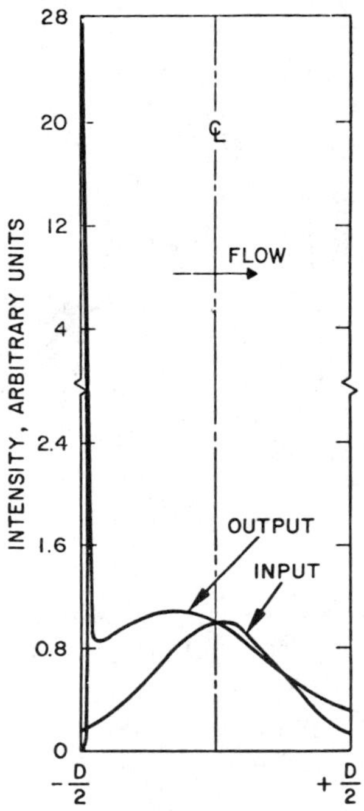

FIG. 10.11

FIG. 10.10 Gasdynamic laser gain distributions with and without power extraction.

FIG. 10.11 Geometric optics calculation of intensity distribution over the laser beam for a gasdynamic laser amplifier. (After Clark, 1972.)

beam. Such a nonuniform gain profile ultimately leads to a nonuniform intensity variation across the output beam. This variation is shown in Fig. 10.11, obtained from Clark (1972). Here the intensity distribution of the input beam in a MOPA (a Gaussian profile) is compared with the corresponding output intensity distribution. Note that the upstream edge of the output beam (where gain is high) peaks to a very high value. These results clearly show the nonuniformity of the output beam as caused by a nonuniform gain profile.

The results shown in Fig. 10.11 were computed based on geometric optics. However, in the region of peak intensity on the upstream side, diffraction is important. Figure 10.12, also obtained from Clark (1972), shows the same case except that a more complicated, physical optics calculation is used to obtain the output intensity distribution. The effect of diffraction

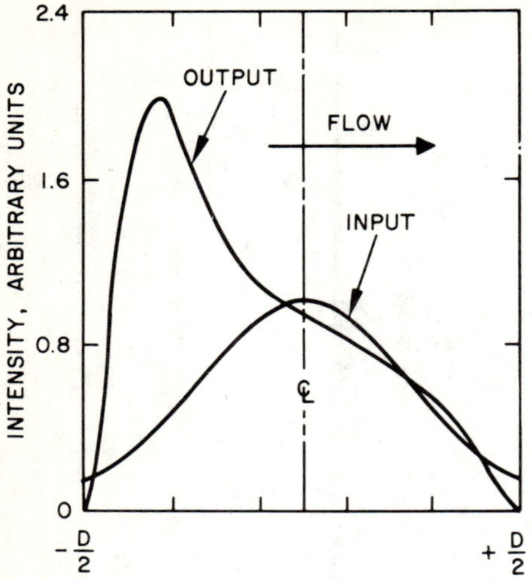

FIG. 10.12 Physical optics calculation of intensity distribution over the laser beam for the gasdynamic laser amplifier of Fig. 10.11. (After Clark, 1972.)

is to smooth out the sharpness of the peak as predicted from geometric optics in Fig. 10.11. However, Fig. 10.12 still shows a very nonuniform intensity distribution across the beam.

The amount of power contained in a focused beam in the far field does not seem to be materially reduced by a nonuniform distribution in the near field. However, the peak levels of the nonuniform intensity distribution may cause local overheating of the cavity output mirror or window, which could cause major problems. Therefore, such nonuniform peaks as shown in Fig. 10.12 must be accounted for in mirror and window design.

Chapter XI

Aerodynamic Windows

11.1 Introduction

As discussed in Chapter X, the laser beam extracted from a gasdynamic laser may have a nonuniform intensity distribution, and the local intensity may peak to very large values (see, for example, Figs. 10.11 and 10.12). Therefore, there may be local heating rates on the cavity mirrors or windows that can be high enough to cause loss of optical quality at the very least or total material failure at the worst. In the face of this problem, how do we physically extract the high intensity laser beam from the cavity and allow it to pass to the surrounding atmosphere? One technique was mentioned in Chapters IV and V, namely, to have a number of holes in a water-cooled output mirror through which a portion of the radiation can pass. This is effective in extracting raw power but causes major problems with beam quality. Incidentally, air leaks from the outside into the cavity through these holes can have a deleterious effect on the supersonic flow in the cavity and diffuser.

An alternative technique is simply to extract the beam through a solid window. However, as mentioned above, a certain amount of the laser energy is always absorbed by the window material, and for high energy lasers the window heating causes a rapid deterioration of its transparency. In fact, at present there are no existing solid windows for practical use on high energy lasers.

A third technique, and the one that is most viable for present high energy lasers of all types—electrical, chemical, and gasdynamic—is to extract the beam through an *aerodynamic window*. The basic principle of an aerodynamic window is as follows. The pressure in a gasdynamic laser cavity is typically on the order of 0.05 to 0.1 atm, considerably less than the 1 atm existing outside the laser at sea level. Therefore, any mechanism used to physically extract the laser beam from the cavity must somehow support this large pressure difference across the output aperture. An aerodynamic window is a device that creates such an interface between the low pressure cavity and the high pressure surroundings by purely gasdynamic means, using a stream of gas that is transparent to the laser radiation. In this fashion the laser beam can exit from the cavity without causing the material problems discussed above.

Parmentier (1972) has performed a systematic study of aerodynamic windows that employ supersonic flow across the aperture. The following sections draw from his results.

11.2 Concepts

Consider a supersonic flow along a flat surface, as shown in Fig. 11.1. The static pressure is p_1. If the surface is deflected downward at a corner as shown at the top of Fig. 11.1, an expansion wave is created that decreases the static pressure. Likewise, if the surface is deflected upward at a corner as shown at the bottom of Fig. 11.1, an oblique shock wave is created that increases the static pressure. Hence expansion and shock waves can clearly act as a boundary between the pressure inside the cavity of a GDL and the ambient pressure of the surroundings.

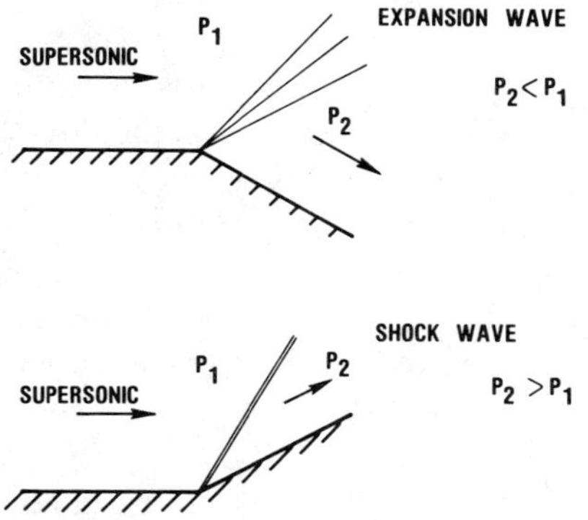

FIG. 11.1 Pressure changes across shock and expansion waves.

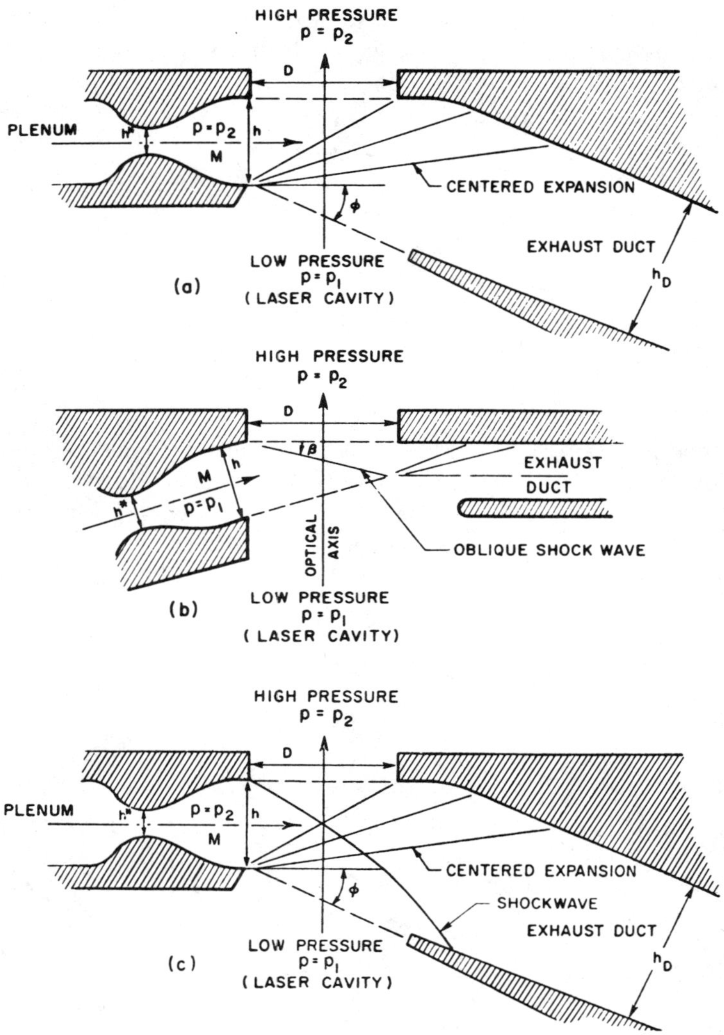

FIG. 11.2 Various types of supersonic flow aerodynamic windows. (After Parmentier, 1972.)

This is the underlying idea of the aerodynamic windows discussed by Parmentier (1972), which are shown in Fig. 11.2. Here, three types of windows are illustrated. All three use a convergent–divergent nozzle to expand the flow to supersonic speeds. In the expansion window an expansion wave is formed at the nozzle lip on the cavity side. In the compression window an oblique shock wave is formed at the nozzle lip on the ambient side. The shock–expansion window combines both of the above wave systems. In all three the laser beam propagates out of the low pressure cavity, through the expansion and/or shock waves, and into the ambient air at 1 atm. Since air is almost transparent at 10.6 μm, the laser intensity is not attenuated. Of course, with the aerodynamic window, there are no material heating problems.

11.3 Results

Parmentier (1972) has carried out theoretical calculations and laboratory experiments validating the aerodynamic window concepts shown in Fig. 11.2. However, he also underscores a drawback of such windows, namely, that they require high mass flow rates of dry air or N_2. This mass flow is proportional to the square of the aperture diameter D (see Fig.

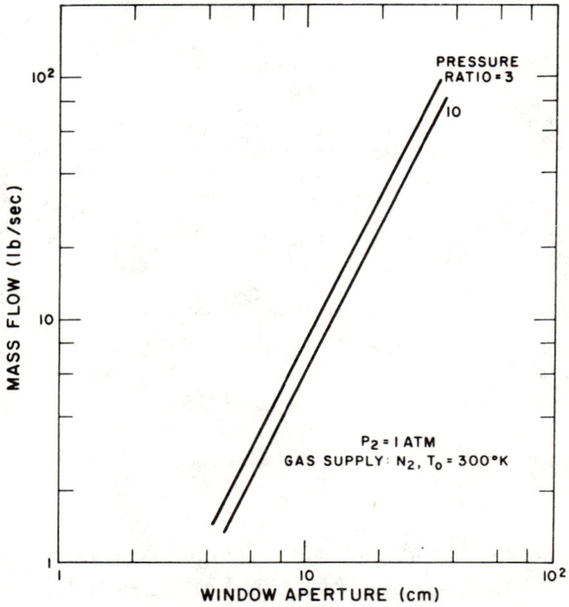

FIG. 11.3 Mass flow required for compression window operation. (After Parmentier, 1972.)

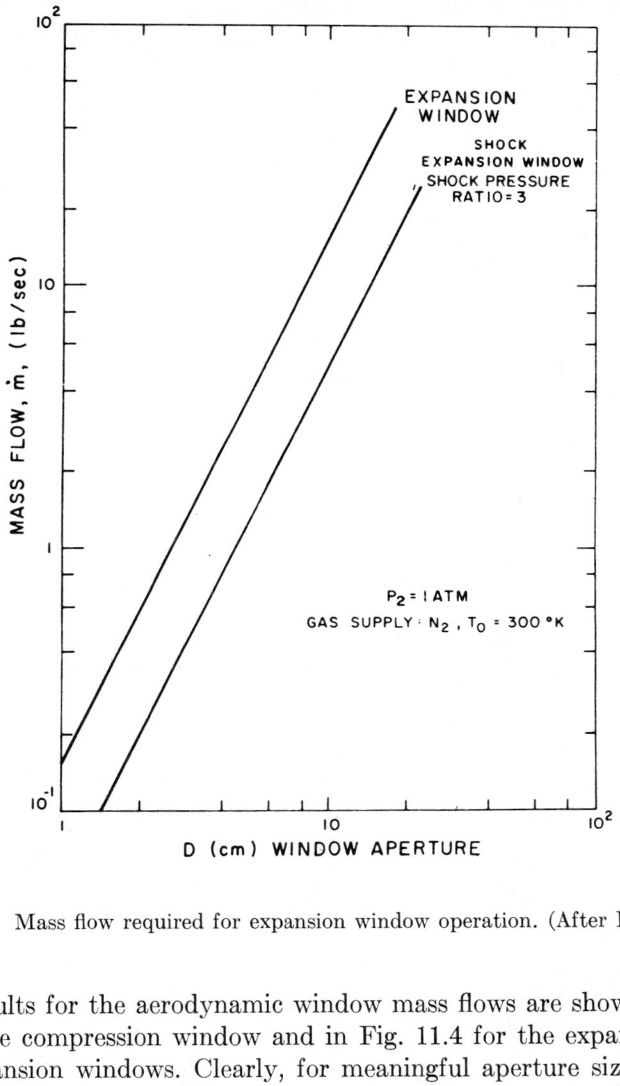

FIG. 11.4 Mass flow required for expansion window operation. (After Parmentier, 1972.)

11.2). Results for the aerodynamic window mass flows are shown in Fig. 11.3 for the compression window and in Fig. 11.4 for the expansion and shock–expansion windows. Clearly, for meaningful aperture sizes on the order of 10 to 20 cm, large mass flow rates are required. Parmentier (1972) points out that the shock–expansion window requires the smallest mass flow of any of the three types.

There are density variations in the beam direction through these aerodynamic windows; hence there are phase distortions introduced into the beam by the window. For the expansion or compression windows the phase distortion is linear, resulting in simple beam shearing but no degradation in the far field. The density distributions through a shock-expansion window calculated by the method of characteristics are given by Parmentier (1972) and are shown in Fig. 11.5. The corresponding phase distortion is shown in Fig. 11.6.

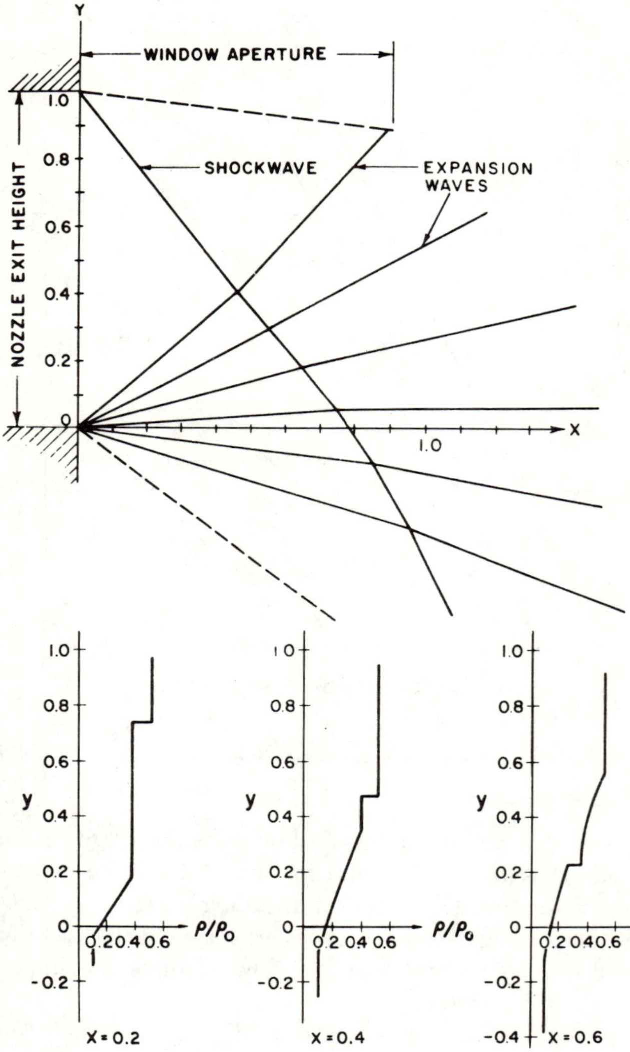

FIG. 11.5 Calculated wave structure and density field in the shock-expansion window aperture. (After Parmentier, 1972.)

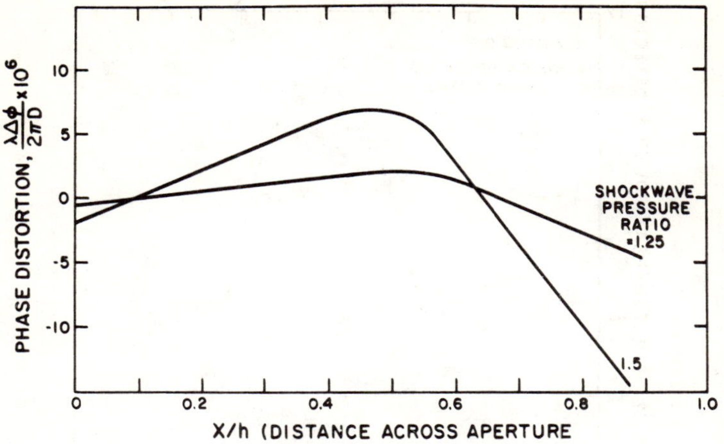

FIG. 11.6 Nondimensional phase variation across the output aperture. (After Parmentier, 1972.)

Parmentier (1972) has conducted experiments with a shock–expansion window. Among these tests an independent CO_2 laser beam from an electric discharge laser was passed through a 4-cm aperture aerodynamic window, as shown in Fig. 11.7. The results for the output beam intensity distribu-

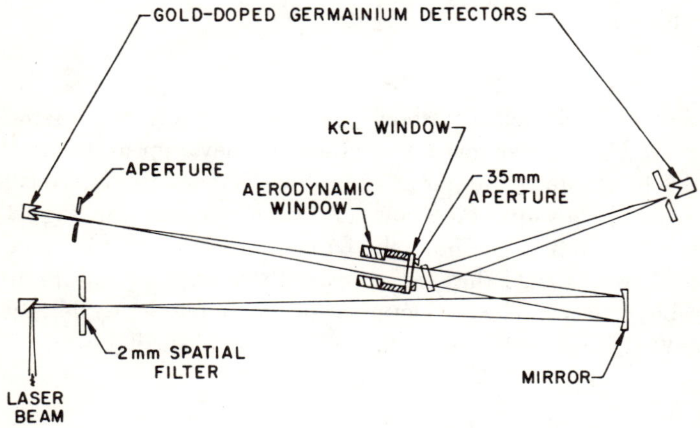

FIG. 11.7 Optical system for measuring beam quality degradation. (After Parmentier, 1972.)

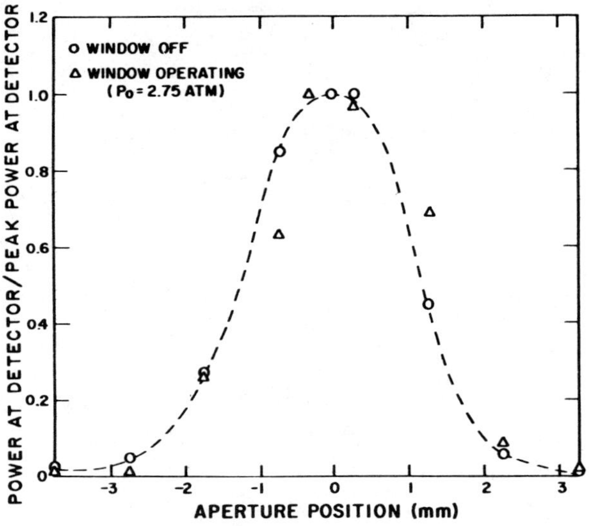

FIG. 11.8 Intensity distributions obtained by moving the scanning aperture through the focal point. (After Parmentier, 1972.)

tion are shown in Fig. 11.8, which indicates only a small effect of the flow on the beam.

11.4 Summary

The above results clearly show the feasibility of using aerodynamic windows on high power gas lasers. Indeed, they appear to be the only practical solution until a major advancement is made in materials for solid windows. Also, the supersonic flows and concepts shown in Figs. 11.1 and 11.2 are by no means the only fluid dynamic concepts for aerodynamic windows. Any flow field that can support the required pressure difference is a possible concept. The development of aerodynamic windows is still in its infancy; there is much work still to be accomplished.

Chapter XII

Diffusers

12.1 Introduction

As stated in Chapter I, gasdynamic lasers are essentially supersonic wind tunnels. As a result, they share many of the same aerodynamic problems that have been encountered over the years with the development of supersonic and hypersonic wind tunnels: for example, the attainment of proper reservoir conditions; the proper contouring of the supersonic expansion nozzles for parallel, uniform flow; the minimization of the adverse effects of boundary layers and shock waves; and the design of an efficient diffuser downstream of the test section or cavity. Basic information regarding these matters can be found in most textbooks on compressible flow, such as those by Liepmann and Roshko (1957) and Shapiro (1953), and therefore are beyond the scope of this book. However, for reasons described below, diffusers for gasdynamic lasers are somewhat different from those used by supersonic wind tunnels. Moreover, to the author's knowledge, every existing practical gasdynamic laser that exhausts directly to the atmosphere has had its share of diffuser problems. For these reasons, this chapter gives a short presentation of phenomena associated with gasdynamic laser diffusers. Also, because the diffuser is physically located at the end of a gasdynamic laser, it seems fitting that the end of this book be devoted to its discussion.

12.2 Purpose of the Diffuser

Figure 1.1 in Chapter I shows a schematic of the principal CO_2–N_2 gasdynamic laser hardware components for the flowing gas, including the diffuser. The gas starts out in the reservoir with pressure p_0, flows through the nozzles and cavity where the static pressure drops to a low subatmospheric value, and then is exhausted to the atmosphere after passing through the diffuser. The job of the diffuser is to decrease the flow velocity from high supersonic to low subsonic speeds, increasing its pressure up to ambient pressure, with a minimum of dissipative losses. That is, a diffuser is designed to recover as much of the original total pressure of the flow p_0 as possible. Dissipative phenomena, namely shock waves and boundary layer viscous effects, work against this recovery, and the pressure at the exit of the diffuser p_e is always less than p_0. The ratio p_0/p_e is defined as the tunnel pressure ratio; it is always greater than one, but the job of the diffuser is to make it as low as nature allows.

Experience has shown that an efficient supersonic diffuser has the general shape as shown in Fig. 12.1. The entrance section is a gently converging duct with angle θ_1, followed by a constant area section of length L_d. The flow enters supersonically, and, owing to the action of oblique shock waves and the boundary layer, the velocity is slowed to a near sonic value at the end of the constant area duct. The divergent section with angle θ_2 is a subsonic diffuser, which further slows the velocity to a low subsonic value before it is exhausted to the atmosphere. The entrance area, the area of the straight duct, and the exit area are designated A_1, A_2, and A_3, respectively.

The proper design of this diffuser, i.e., proper values for θ_1, θ_2, L_d, and A_1/A_2, depends critically on the entrance Mach number, the Reynolds number, and the flow field structure entering the diffuser. *There are no pat answers.* It is important to accept the fact that contemporary supersonic and hypersonic diffuser design is more of an *art* than a science. This is particularly true for the CO_2–N_2 gasdynamic laser diffuser because of its

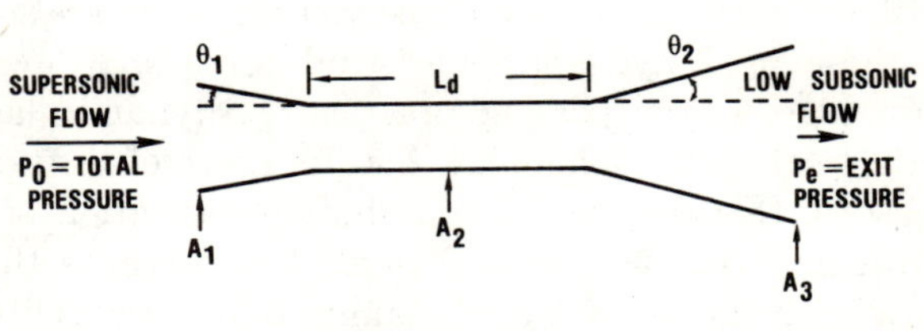

FIG. 12.1 Supersonic diffuser.

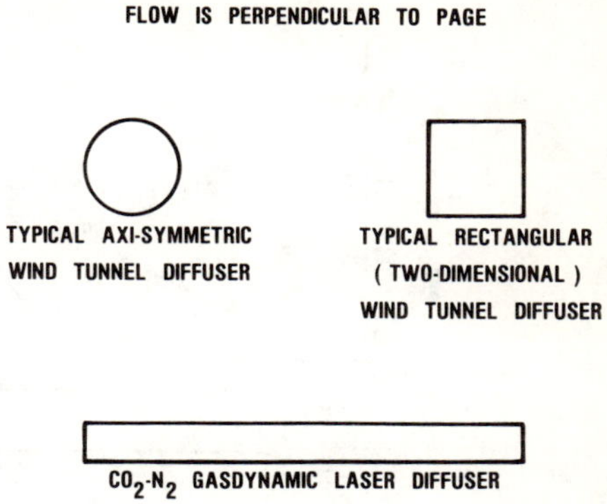

FIG. 12.2 Contrast between wind tunnel and gasdynamic laser diffuser cross sections.

"high aspect ratio" cross section, i.e., a long, thin rectangle. This is shown in Fig. 12.2, where the gasdynamic laser diffuser cross section is contrasted with those for typical supersonic wind tunnels. The flow can be visualized as moving perpendicular to the page. Moreover, referring again to Fig. 1.1, the multinozzle flow in a gasdynamic laser leads to multiple wakes and weak oblique shock systems entering the diffuser. Such a flow is not characteristic of typical supersonic wind tunnels. For these reasons gasdynamic laser diffuser design is relatively unique, and hence, in this case, there is even more emphasis on the art rather than the science.

12.3 Diffuser Flow Field

The uncertainties in supersonic diffuser design are caused mainly by the complex flow field structure inside the device. The flow field is characterized by a complicated interaction between oblique shock waves and the wall boundary layer. The flow may separate from the wall where the shock waves

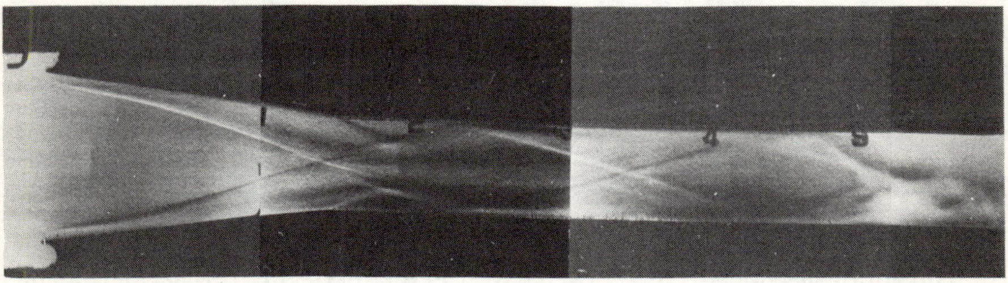

FIG. 12.3 Schlieren photograph of the flow in a two-dimensional supersonic diffuser.

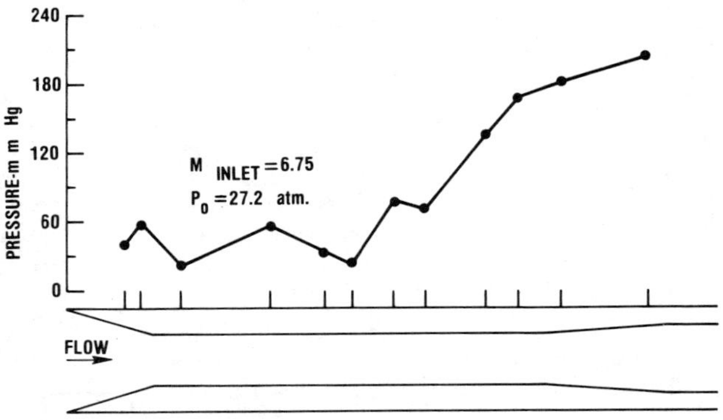

FIG. 12.4 Static pressure distribution along the wall of a supersonic diffuser.

impinge on the boundary layer. The adverse pressure gradient, i.e., the increasing static pressure in the flow direction inside the diffuser, will also promote flow separation.

These characteristics are clearly shown in Figs. 12.3 and 12.4, taken from some previously unpublished diffuser research work of the present author. Figure 12.3 is a schlieren photograph of the flow in a two-dimensional supersonic diffuser. The entrance Mach number is 7, and flow is from left to right. Note the oblique shock waves emanating from the lip of the diffuser entrance and the multiple interaction and intersection of these shocks downstream, forming a typical diamond shock pattern. The pattern dissipates downstream, and a weak normal shock wave is barely visible far downstream. Figure 12.4 illustrates the wall static pressure variation along the diffuser. Note that the pressure first alternately increases and decreases, a ramification of the alternate compression–expansion regions present in the constant area section. Then, downstream of the region where the diamond shock pattern dissipates, the static pressure increases considerably. Clearly Figs. 12.3 and 12.4 indicate a very complex flow within the diffuser. As a result, accurate aerodynamic calculations of this flow still remain to be accomplished. *This is why diffuser design is still an empirical procedure.*

12.4 Normal Shock Recovery

The simplest conceptual shock pattern in a supersonic diffuser is that of a standing normal shock wave followed by a divergent duct, as shown in

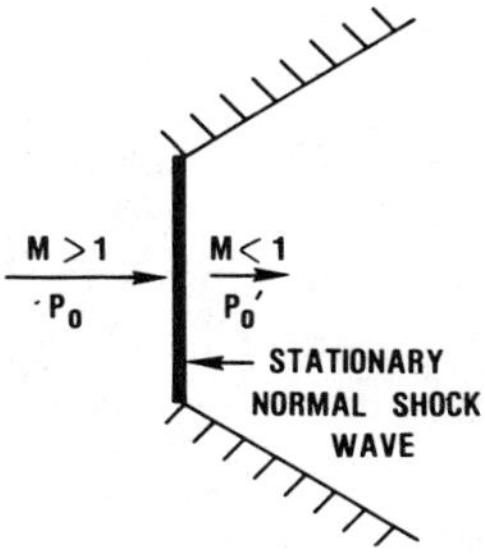

FIG. 12.5 Normal shock wave standing at the entrance of a subsonic diffuser (divergent duct).

Fig. 12.5. There is a loss in total pressure across the normal shock; i.e., $p_0'/p_0 < 1$. Referring again to Fig. 12.3, the flow in an actual supersonic diffuser is obviously much more complicated than shown in Fig. 12.5. However, experience has shown that the pressure recovery through the diffuser shown in Fig. 12.3 is usually close to normal shock recovery. That is, $(p_e/p_0) \approx (p_0'/p_0)$. In fact, it is common to define a diffuser efficiency based on normal shock recovery as

$$\eta_D = (p_e/p_0)/(p_0'/p_0) \tag{12.1}$$

Hopefully, a well-designed supersonic diffuser will yield values of $\eta_D > 1$.

For a calorically perfect gas, p_0'/p_0 is a well-defined function of upstream Mach number M. In turn, the tunnel pressure ratio p_0/p_e will also depend on the cavity Mach number. In Fig. 12.6 normal shock values for the inverse of p_0'/p_0 are shown as the solid curve. The shaded region in Fig. 12.6 gives a semiquantitative picture of the tunnel pressure ratios encountered in practice in supersonic diffusers. It can be seen that normal shock recovery yields a reasonable estimate for the required tunnel pressure ratio.

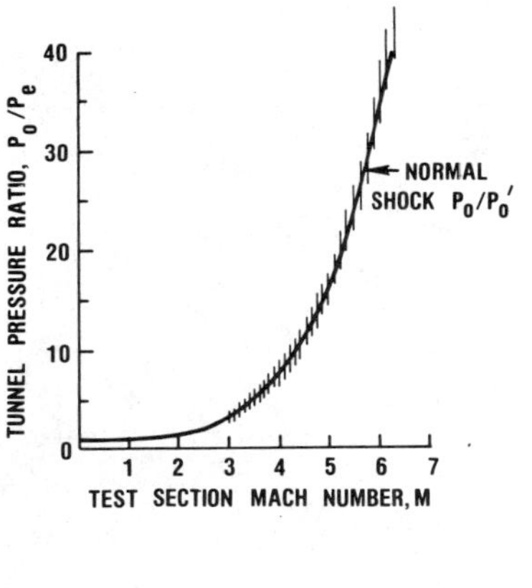

FIG. 12.6 Tunnel pressure ratio as a function of Mach number; experience compared to normal shock recovery.

12.5 Area Ratio

Referring again to Fig. 12.1, probably the most important parameter in supersonic diffuser design is the area ratio A_2/A_1. If we consider a given flow entering a variable geometry diffuser where A_2/A_1 is continuously reduced below unity, η_D will first increase, reach a peak value (for A_2/A_1 on the order of 0.4 to 0.5), and then drop suddenly as A_2/A_1 is reduced below a certain critical minimum. This behavior is shown schematically for a typical hypersonic diffuser in Fig. 12.7. When A_2/A_1 is less than the value shown by the vertical dashed line, the flow is choked; i.e., the diffuser throat area A_2 is too small to pass the mass flow issuing from the nozzles. When the diffuser chokes, the supersonic flow field in the laser cavity and possibly in the nozzles themselves will break down. It is important to note that the area ratio for maximum η_D is close to that for choking. Hence an efficient supersonic diffuser will have as small as possible value for A_2/A_1—but not too small.

There is another important consideration associated with the diffuser area ratio. Consider the flow through a supersonic tunnel when it is first started. The starting process will invariably include unsteady shock waves in the nozzles and cavity. As the steady flow establishes itself, these unsteady shock waves are swept downstream and must be "swallowed" by the diffuser. In turn, the diffuser throat area A_2 must be large enough to pass the shock waves. Unfortunately, this value of A_2 required to "start the diffuser" is always larger than the value for peak efficiency. The area ratio for starting is shown schematically as the solid vertical line in Fig. 12.7. *Therefore, in the design of a fixed-geometry diffuser, the value chosen for* A_2/A_1

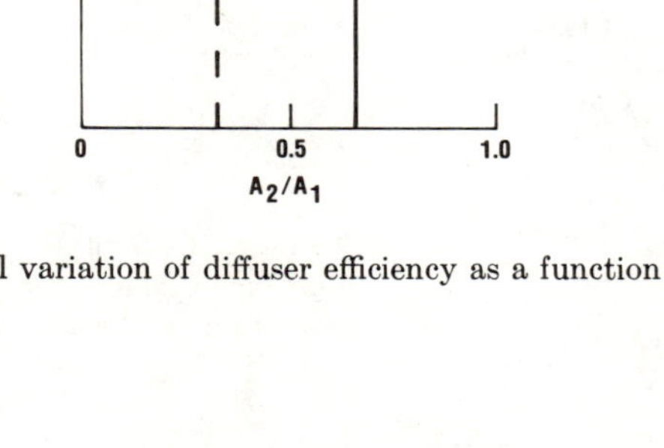

FIG. 12.7 Typical variation of diffuser efficiency as a function of diffuser throat to inlet area ratio.

must not be less than that required to start the flow. As a result, fixed-geometry diffusers have design area ratios that are too large to achieve the peak value of η_D shown in Fig. 12.7. This also demonstrates the value of variable-geometry diffusers where A_2 changes during the run. In such a variable-geometry device, A_2/A_1 is initially large enough to start the flow and then is contracted to the smaller value to obtain peak η_D. Variable-geometry diffusers are usually complicated mechanical designs, especially with regard to providing seals against leaks from the outside. For this reason, almost all existing supersonic and hypersonic wind tunnels have fixed-geometry diffusers. All practical gasdynamic lasers to date have also used fixed-geometry designs.

In a two-dimensional, supersonic wind tunnel where the area of the throat of the supersonic nozzle is A^* and the nozzle exit area is A_1, the same as the diffuser entrance area, then an approximate design formula for the minimum diffuser area ratio required for starting is

$$A_2/A_1 = (A^*/A_1)/(p_0'/p_0) \tag{12.2}$$

where p_0'/p_0 is calculated from the cavity Mach number. This equation is obtained from simple one-dimensional gasdynamic relations and calculates the A_2 required to pass the mass flow behind a normal shock wave standing at the diffuser entrance. It does not account for the real starting shock process, nor does it include viscous boundary layer effects. Therefore, Eq. (12.2) is approximate. Particularly for the high aspect ratio diffusers for gasdynamic lasers, Eq. (12.2) should be viewed simply as an educated guess. This is partly because the ratio of wetted surface area to cross-section area is much larger for gasdynamic lasers diffusers than for conventional wind tunnel diffusers, hence accentuating the boundary layer effects.

12.6 Drop-Out Pressure

Consider a fixed-geometry diffuser with A_2/A_1 equal to or larger than the minimum required for starting. A certain tunnel pressure ratio p_0/p_e is required for starting the flow. However, experience has shown that once the starting shocks have been swallowed by the diffuser and steady flow is attained through the wind tunnel, the tunnel pressure ratio can actually be decreased without "unstarting" the flow. The lowest value to which p_0/p_e can be decreased without destroying the flow is called the drop-out pressure ratio. This phenomenon is illustrated in Fig. 12.8, which compares

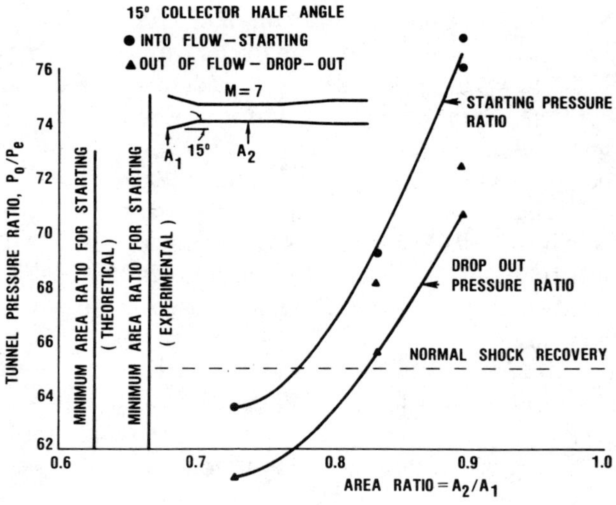

FIG. 12.8 Variation of starting and drop-out pressure ratios with diffuser throat to inlet area ratio.

data for starting and drop-out pressure ratios versus diffuser area ratio for a cavity Mach number of 7. Note that, for these conditions, the tunnel pressure ratio can be reduced by 5 to 8% after the flow has started. The same phenomenon is seen in Fig. 12.9 versus diffuser entrance angle θ_1. The sensitivity of diffuser efficiency to θ_1 is also apparant from Fig. 12.9.

These results indicate that a hard-to-start diffuser may be set into flow by overpressuring, i.e., by starting the flow with a pressure pulse and then

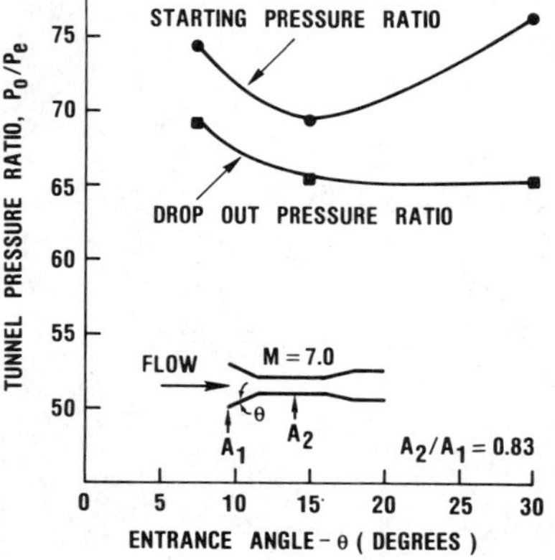

FIG. 12.9 Variation of starting and drop-out pressure ratios with diffuser inlet ramp angle.

decreasing the tunnel pressure ratio to the desired conditions. This technique has been successful in some wind tunnels and gasdynamic lasers.

12.7 Summary

Emphasis is again made that diffuser design is more of an art than a science. Some of the phenomena associated with supersonic diffusers have been discussed here, and general comments with regard to configuration and operating conditions have been made. However, these should be construed only as examples. There are many "tricks of the trade," and the reader should inform himself of these tricks before embarking on a serious diffuser design. Moreover, all pertinent experimental data should be examined. Diffuser design is empirical; experimental data and experience must be incorporated in any new configuration.

Appendix A

Effect of Uncertainties in the Kinetic Rates

In the text many comparisons have been made between experiment and theory for CO_2–N_2 gasdynamic lasers. Fair agreement has been obtained in some, but not all, cases. With the rapid development of such lasers, there is an increasing need to obtain closer agreement between prediction and experiment; indeed, it is desirable to calculate gasdynamic laser performance as accurately as possible—ultimately to within a few percent.

At present there is an inherent limitation to the accuracy with which such calculations can be made, namely, the uncertainty in the pertinent vibrational kinetic rates. The heart of a gasdynamic laser is the nonequilibrium nozzle expansion, in which the population inversion is created, and the laser cavity downstream of the nozzle exit, where power is extracted. In both these regions the computed nonequilibrium flow (and hence the theoretical laser performance) is dependent on a complex finite-rate vibrational energy exchange mechanism that is still not yet fully understood. For the CO_2–N_2–H_2O mixture common to most gasdynamic lasers, at least eight distinct vibrational kinetic rates must be utilized in the calculations. In turn, uncertainties in these rates will cause inaccuracies in the computed gasdynamic laser performance. Hence two questions immediately arise: (1) What are the present uncertainties in the measured kinetic rates, and (2) how sensitive are calculations of gasdynamic laser performance to these uncertainties?

This appendix describes some numerical experiments carried out in order to test the sensitivity of gasdynamic laser gain and maximum available energy in the laser cavity to uncertainties in the kinetic rates. These calculations were made with an existing computer program developed by Glowacki and Anderson (1971). This computer code is based on the time-dependent nonequilibrium nozzle flow analysis discussed in Chapter IV.

The vibrational kinetic rates pertinent to CO_2–N_2 gas lasers were examined and compiled by Taylor and Bitterman, first in 1967 and slightly updated in 1969. These references are timely and excellent surveys and have become a standard source for laser calculations. However, Taylor and Bitterman (1969) clearly show that a large scatter existed in much of the data; moreover, for a few rates, only one set of data were available. Anderson (1973, 1974) has compiled additional CO_2–N_2–H_2O vibrational rates measured or calculated since 1969 and has compared these recent data with the standard Taylor and Bitterman data. Moreover, an effort has been made to assess uncertainties that currently exist in these rates.

The reactions that must be included in the calculation of small-signal gain and maximum available energy in gasdynamic lasers are:

1. $CO_2^*(\nu_2) + H_2O \rightleftarrows CO_2 + H_2O$
2. $N_2^* + H_2O \rightleftarrows N_2 + H_2O$
3. $CO_2^*(\nu_3) + H_2O \rightleftarrows CO_2^{***}(\nu_2) + H_2O$
4. $CO_2^*(\nu_2) + N_2 \rightleftarrows CO_2 + N_2$
5. $CO_2^*(\nu_2) + CO_2 \rightleftarrows 2CO_2$
6. $CO_2^*(\nu_3) + N_2 \rightleftarrows CO_2^{***}(\nu_2) + N_2$
7. $CO_2^*(\nu_3) + CO_2 \rightleftarrows CO_2^{***}(\nu_2) + CO_2$
8. $N_2^* + N_2 \rightleftarrows 2N_2$

For calculations, the pumping rate between excited N_2 and $CO_2(001)$, as well as the Fermi resonance between $CO_2(100)$ and $CO_2(020)$, are considered to be sufficiently rapid that local equilibrium is established between N_2 and CO_2 (ν_3) as well as between CO_2 (ν_1) and CO_2 (ν_2). Hence the rates for these reactions are not considered here. However, as discussed in Chapter III, recent information has raised some questions about the local equilibrium normally assumed between the CO_2 (ν_1) and CO_2 (ν_2) modes.

The computer code of Glowacki and Anderson (1971) is used to calculate gasdynamic laser gain G_0 and maximum available energy e_{max} as a function of reservoir temperature T_0. Results are obtained for both a typical first-generation gasdynamic laser (nozzle exit to throat area ratio $A_e/A^* = 20$, reservoir pressure $p_0 = 20$ atm, throat height $h^* = 1$ mm, and mole fractions X_{CO_2} and X_{H_2O} equal to 0.07 and 0.01, respectively), and a second-generation laser ($A_e/A^* = 50$, $p_0 = 37.5$ atm, $h^* = 0.365$ mm, $X_{CO_2} =$

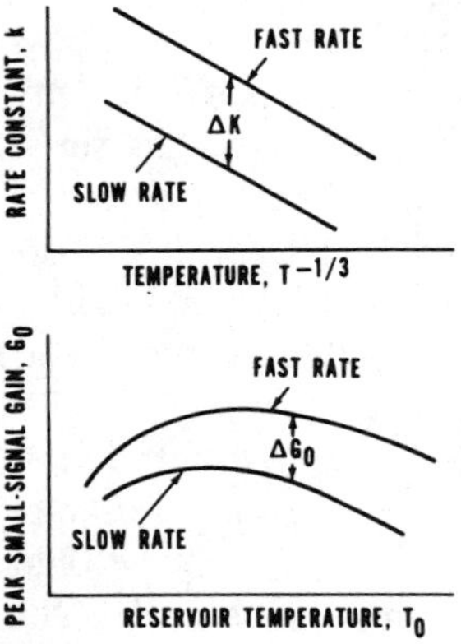

FIG. A.1 Sketch defining parameters used in the numerical experiments.

0.07, $X_{H_2O} = 0.035$). Calculations were made alternately employing fast and slow rates for each kinetic reaction, one at a time. These rates are shown schematically at the top of Fig. A.1. The vertical distance between the slow and fast rate constants k defines a "change in rate constant," Δk. In turn, this change Δk causes a corresponding change in small-signal gain G_0, as shown at the bottom of Fig. A.1. Hence a *sensitivity factor* S can be defined for each rate as

$$S = (\Delta G_0/G_0)/(\Delta k/k)$$

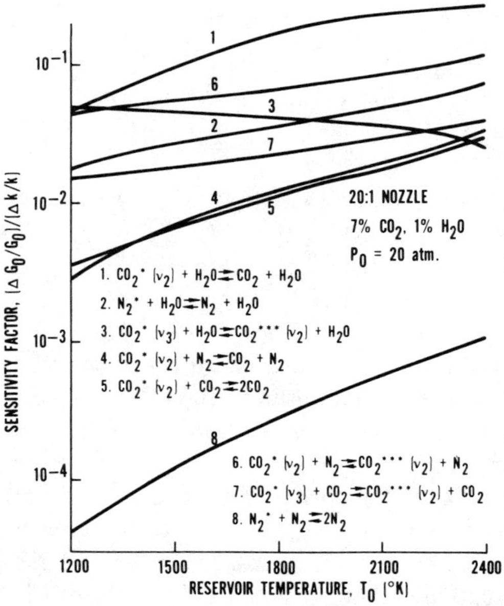

FIG. A.2 Gain sensitivity factor; first-generation gasdynamic laser.

Therefore, *S physically represents the uncertainty in gain per unit uncertainty in rate constant.* The actual values used for Δk along with the resulting G_0 for each kinetic reaction are detailed by Anderson (1973, 1974); hence only the resulting sensitivity factors will be discussed here.

Considering maximum available energy $e_{\max}$, a sensitivity factor can also be defined analogous to that for gain. This factor is shown in Figs. A.4 and A.5 for the first- and second-generation laser cases, respectively. Curves for the rates involving deactivation of the lower laser level are not shown because they have a minimal effect on $e_{\max}$. Comparing Figs. A.4 and A.5 with A.2 and A.3, the reactions that exert maximum and minimum sensitivities on $e_{\max}$ are the same as those that exert maximum and minimum sensitivity on G_0.

The results shown in Figs. A.2 to A.5 are uncertainties in performance *per unit uncertainty in rate constant,* hence they indicate the *sensitivity* of gasdynamic laser calculations to the individual rates. However, some rate constants are known more accurately than others. Hence the question is now posed: What are the absolute uncertainties in G_0 and $e_{\max}$ due to the existing absolute uncertainties in rate constants? Some absolute uncertainties are given below and were obtained from examination of the data scatter shown by Anderson (1973, 1974).

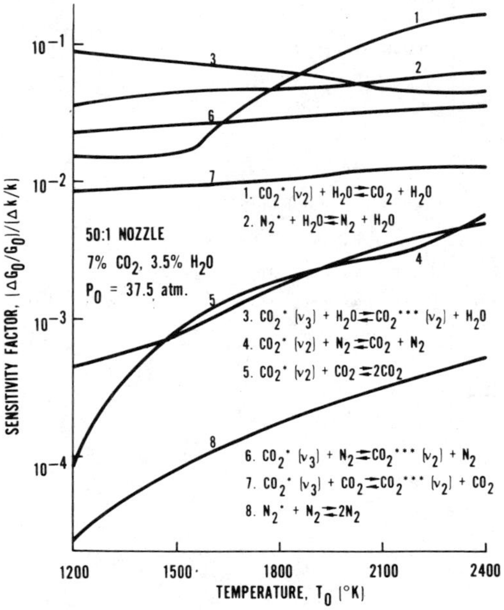

FIG. A.3 Gain sensitivity factor; second-generation gasdynamic laser.

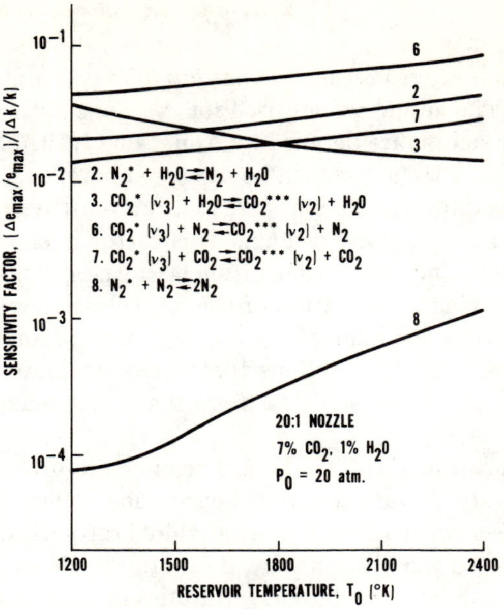

FIG. A.4 Maximum available energy sensitivity factor; first-generation gasdynamic laser.

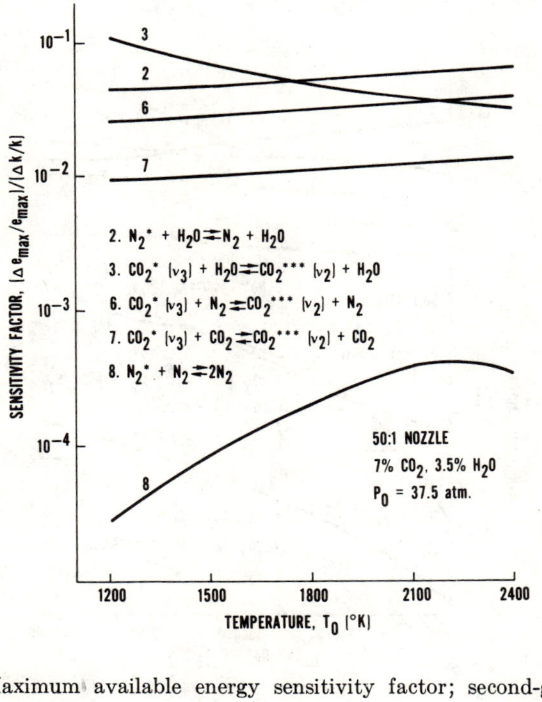

FIG. A.5 Maximum available energy sensitivity factor; second-generation gasdynamic laser.

Reaction	*Uncertainty in data, $\Delta k/k$*
1. $CO_2^*(\nu_2) + H_2O \rightleftarrows CO_2 + H_2O$	3
2. $N_2^* + H_2O \rightleftarrows N_2 + H_2O$	5
3. $CO_2^*(\nu_3) + H_2O \rightleftarrows CO_2^{***}(\nu_2) + H_2O$	5
4. $CO_2^*(\nu_2) + N_2 \rightleftarrows CO_2 + N_2$	4
5. $CO_2^*(\nu_2) + CO_2 \rightleftarrows 2CO_2$	0.5
6. $CO_2^*(\nu_3) + N_2 \rightleftarrows CO_2^{***}(\nu_2) + N_2$	5.0
7. $CO_2^*(\nu_3) + CO_2 \rightleftarrows CO_2^{***}(\nu_2) + CO_2$	0.25
8. $N_2^* + N_2 \rightleftarrows 2N_2$	0.5

These uncertainties are subjective judgments. They are obtained by comparing old and new data from the existing literature, with no particular knowledge of which data may be more valid than the other. Hence the above values of $\Delta k/k$ are probably conservative and do not represent the real uncertainties that exist today. The real uncertainties are probably less than shown above. Nevertheless, they are useful to establish some upper bounds.

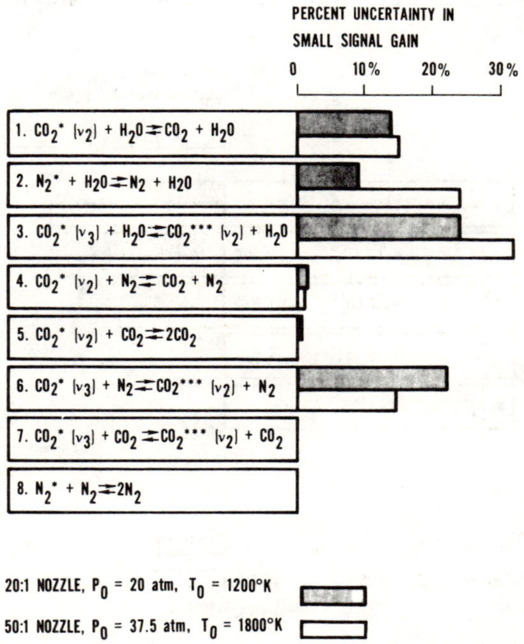

FIG. A.6 Some upper bounds on uncertainty in small-signal gain.

When the sensitivity factors shown in Figs. A.2 to A.5 are multiplied by the above absolute rate data uncertainties $\Delta k/k$, overall uncertainties in G_0 and e_{max} are obtained. These results are shown as bar charts in Figs. A.6 and A.7 for G_0 and e_{max}, respectively. In these figures reservoir temperatures of 1200 and 1800°K are chosen as typical of first- and second-generation gasdynamic lasers, respectively. Note from Figs. A.6 and A.7 that the maximum absolute uncertainties are on the order of 30%. *The reader should construe this only as some measure of an upper bound; as discussed above, the true uncertainty is most likely smaller.*

In the above results the kinetic rates were changed one at a time in order to isolate their individual influence on the calculations. In order to examine the combined effect of rate uncertainties, two additional calculations are made wherein, first, all slow rates are used simultaneously, and alternately, all fast rates are used. The fast and slow rates for these calculations were obtained from the absolute uncertainties $\Delta k/k$ listed above, centered around a mean reference value given by the reference rates (or relaxation times) quoted in Appendix B. The results are given in Fig. A.8 for small-signal gain as a function of T_0. Again, these results should be interpreted as very conservative bounds; the real uncertainty is probably much less.

From the above study of the sensitivity of gasdynamic laser gain and maximum available energy to uncertainties in the vibrational rate data,

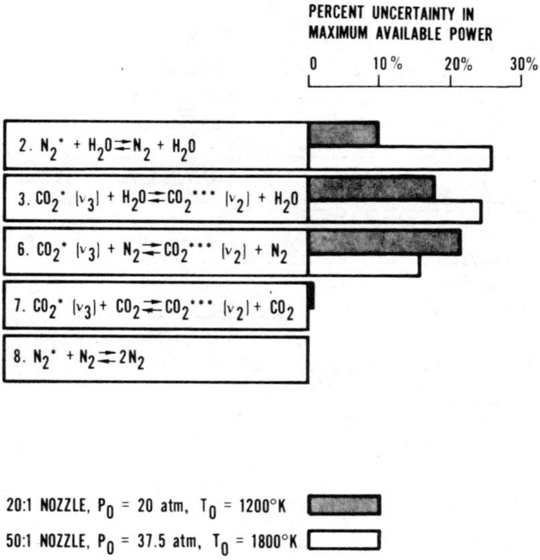

FIG. A.7 Some upper bounds on uncertainty in maximum available energy in the laser cavity.

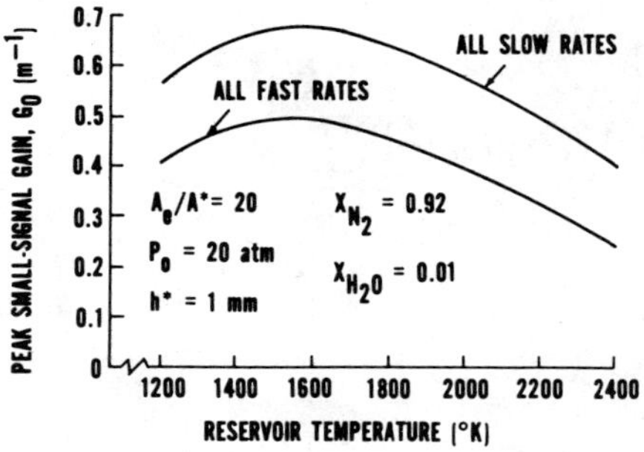

FIG. A.8 Uncertainties in gain bounded by simultaneously all fast rates and simultaneously all slow rates.

the following conclusions are made:

(1) The calculated results are most sensitive to the following processes:

$$CO_2^*(\nu_2) + H_2O \rightleftarrows CO_2 + H_2O$$

$$CO_2^*(\nu_3) + H_2O \rightleftarrows CO_2^{***}(\nu_2) + H_2O$$

$$CO_2^*(\nu_3) + N_2 \rightleftarrows CO_2^{***}(\nu_2) + N_2$$

$$N_2^* + H_2O \rightleftarrows N_2 + H_2O$$

It is important that accurate rates, along with their proper temperature dependence, be utilized for these reactions.

(2) At most, gasdynamic laser gain and maximum available energy are uncertain to about 30% owing to the major uncertainties between old and new rate data in the existing literature. In reality, using some insight as to which rates are more valid, the actual uncertainty in gasdynamic laser calculations could be much less.

Appendix B

Vibrational Relaxation Times for the CO_2–N_2–H_2O *or* He *System*

The following approximate correlations are suggested for the relaxation times necessary to calculate gasdynamic laser gain and maximum available power using the techniques described in this book. These correlations have been used to generate the information in Appendix A. The kinetic rate data used to obtain these correlations are a combination of the data presented by Taylor and Bitterman (1967, 1969) and the more recent data compiled by Anderson (1973, 1974).

$$(\tau_a p)_{CO_2\text{–}N_2} = 1.3 \times 10^5 \, (T^{-1/3})^{4.9}$$

$$(\tau_a p)_{CO_2\text{–}CO_2} = 0.27 \, (\tau_a p)_{CO_2\text{–}N_2}$$

$$(\tau_a p)_{CO_2\text{–}H_2O} = 5.5 \times 10^{-2}$$

$$\log(\tau_b p)_{N_2\text{–}N_2} = 93 \, (T^{-1/3}) - 4.61$$

$$(\tau_b p)_{N_2\text{–}CO_2} = (\tau_b p)_{N_2\text{–}N_2}$$

$$\log(\tau_b p)_{N_2\text{–}H_2O} = 27.65 \, (T^{-1/3}) - 3.2415$$

$$\log(\tau_c p)_{CO_2\text{–}CO_2} = 17.8 \, (T^{-1/3}) - 1.808$$

$$(\tau_c p)_{CO_2\text{–}N_2} = 2(\tau_c p)_{CO_2\text{–}CO_2}$$

$$\log(\tau_c p)_{CO_2\text{–}N_2O} = -20.4 \, (T^{-1/3}) + 0.643 \text{ (For } T > 600°\text{K)}$$

$$\log(\tau_c p)_{CO_2\text{–}H_2O} = -20.4 \, (600^{-1/3}) + 0.642$$

$$= \text{const. (for } 200 < T < 600°\text{K)}$$

In the above correlations (τp) is in (μsec-atm) and T is in °K.

Appendix C

The Teare Effect

Consider the local V–V equilibrium between two chemical species such as CO and N_2 discussed in Chapter VIII. The dominant reaction is

$$N_2(v = 1) + CO(v = 0) \underset{k_r}{\overset{k_f}{\rightleftarrows}} N_2(v = 0) + CO(v = 1) \tag{C.1}$$

The corresponding rate equation for the formation of $CO(v = 1)$ is

$$dn_{CO(1)}/dt = k_f n_{N_2(1)} n_{CO(0)} - k_r n_{N_2(0)} n_{CO(1)} \tag{C.2}$$

where k_f and k_r are, by definition, forward and reverse rate constants for the reaction (C.1).

If the gas mixture were in complete thermodynamic equilibrium at the static temperature T, $dn_{CO(1)}/dt = 0$, and Eq. (C.2) gives

$$0 = k_f n_{N_2(1)} n_{CO(0)} - k_r n_{N_2(0)} n_{CO(1)}$$

$$k_f = k_r \frac{n_{N_2(0)}}{n_{N_2(1)}} \frac{n_{CO(1)}}{n_{CO(0)}} = k_r \frac{\exp(-\theta_{CO}/T)}{\exp(-\theta_{N_2}/T)} \tag{C.3}$$

where θ_{CO} and θ_{N_2} are the characteristic vibrational temperatures of CO and N_2, respectively. In Eq. (C.3) the population ratios have been replaced by the Boltzmann distribution at temperature T.

Now assume that the vibrational energies for CO and N_2 are *not* in equilibrium with T but that there exists a *local* V–V equilibrium between CO and N_2. Let $T_v(CO)$ and $T_v(N_2)$ be the vibrational temperatures of CO and N_2, respectively. If the oscillators are harmonic, these vibrational temperatures apply equally to all vibrational energy levels of the given species. If the oscillators are anharmonic, the vibrational temperatures are defined between the $v = 1$ and $v = 0$ levels, as described by Eq. (8.12). For this case of local V–V equilibrium, Eq. (C.2) still holds, and $dn_{CO(1)}/dt$ is still zero. Hence

$$0 = k_f n_{N_2(1)} n_{CO(0)} - k_r n_{N_2(0)} n_{CO(1)} \tag{C.4}$$

However,

$$\frac{n_{N_2(1)}}{n_{N_2(0)}} = \exp[-\theta_{N_2}/T_v(N_2)] \tag{C.5}$$

and

$$\frac{n_{CO(1)}}{n_{CO(0)}} = \exp[-\theta_{CO}/T_v(CO)] \tag{C.6}$$

Substituting Eqs. (C.3), (C.5), and (C.6) into (C.4), we have

$$\exp(-\theta_{CO}/T)/\exp(-\theta_{N_2}/T) = \exp[-\theta_{CO}/T_v(CO)]/\exp[-\theta_{N_2}/T_v(N_2)]$$

or

$$(\theta_{N_2} - \theta_{CO})/T = \theta_{N_2}/T_v(N_2) - \theta_{CO}/T_v(CO) \tag{C.7}$$

Solving (C.7) for $T_v(CO)$, we have

$$T_v(CO) = \theta_{CO}/\{[\theta_{N_2}/T_v(N_2)] - [(\theta_{N_2} - \theta_{CO})/T]\} \tag{C.8}$$

This is Eq. (8.13), quoted in Chapter VIII.

References

Anderson, J. D., Jr. (1969). A Time-Dependent Quasi-One-Dimensional Analysis of Population Inversions in an Expanding Gas. NOLTR 69–200, Naval Ordnance Lab., White Oak, Maryland.

Anderson, J. D., Jr. (1970a). A Time-Dependent Analysis for Vibrational and Chemical Nonequilibrium Nozzle Flows. *AIAA J.* **8**, 545–550.

Anderson, J. D., Jr. (1970b). Numerical Experiments Associated with Gas Dynamic Lasers. NOLTR 70–198, Naval Ordnance Lab., White Oak, Maryland.

Anderson, J. D., Jr., (1970c). Time-Dependent Analysis of Population Inversions in an Expanding Gas. *Phys. Fluids* **13**, 1983–1989.

Anderson, J. D., Jr. (1970d). Time-Dependent Solutions of Nonequilibrium Nozzle Flows—A Sequel. *AIAA J.* **8**, 2280–2282.

Anderson, J. D., Jr. (1972a). Effect of Na on CO_2–N_2 Gasdynamic Laser Gain. *J. Appl. Phys.* **43**, 534–536.

Anderson, J. D., Jr. (1972b). Gas Dynamic Lasers: A State-of-the-Art Survey. *NEREM Record* **14**, 180–183.

Anderson, J. D., Jr. (1973). Sensitivity of Gasdynamic Laser Calculations to Uncertainties in Kinetic Rates. Tech. Rep. No. AE 73–2, Dept. of Aerospace Engineering, Univ. of Maryland, College Park, Maryland.

Anderson, J. D., Jr. (1974). The Effect of Kinetic Rate Uncertainties on Gasdynamic Laser Performance. AIAA Paper No. 74–176.

Anderson, J. D., Jr., and Harris, E. L. (1972a). Modern Advances in the Physics of Gasdynamic Lasers. AIAA Paper No. 72–143.

Anderson, J. D., Jr., and Harris, E. L. (1972b). Gasdynamic Laser 2 Years Later. *Laser Focus* **8**, 32–34.

Anderson, J. D., Jr., and Madden, M. T. (1971). Population Inversions behind Normal Shock Waves. *AIAA J.* **9**, 1630–1632.

Anderson, J. D. Jr., and Winkler, E. M. (1971). High Temperature Aerodynamics with Electromagnetic Radiation. *Proc. IEEE* **59**, 651–658.

Anderson, J. D., Jr., Madden, M. T., and Piper, C. H. (1970). Vibrational Population Inversions behind Normal Shock Waves in CO_2–N_2–He Mixtures. NOLTR 70–214, Naval Ordnance Lab., White Oak, Maryland.

Anderson, J. D., Jr., Humphrey, R. L., Vamos, J. S., Plummer, M. J., and Jensen, R. E. (1971a). Population Inversions in an Expanding Gas: Theory and Experiment. NOLTR 71–116, Naval Ordnance Lab., White Oak, Maryland.

Anderson, J. D., Jr., Humphrey, R. L., Vamos, J. S., Plummer, M. J., and Jensen, R. E. (1971b). Population Inversions in an Expanding Gas: Theory and Experiment. *Phys. Fluids* **14**, 2620–2624.

Basov, N. G., and Oraevskii, A. N. (1963). Attainment of Negative Temperatures by Heating and Cooling of a System. *Sov. Phys. JETP* **17**, 1171–1172.

Basov, N. G., Mikhaylov, V. G., Oraevskii, A. N., and Shcheglov, V. A. (1968). Obtaining a Population Inversion of Molecules in a Supersonic Stream of Binary Gas in a Laval Nozzle. *Zh. Tekh. Fiz.* **38**, 2031–2041.

Biriukov, A. S., Dronov, A. P., Kondriavtsev, E. M., and Sobolev, N. N. (1971). Gas Dynamic CO_2–He–N_2 Laser Investigations. *IEEE J. Quantum Electron.* **QE-7**, 388–391.

Borghi, R., and Charpenel, M. (1972). The High Velocity Mixing between Vibrationally Excited Nitrogen and Carbon Dioxide. *Astron. Acta.* **17**, 833–842.

Bronfin, B. R., Boedeker, L. R., and Cheyer, J. P. (1970). Thermal Laser Excitation by Mixing in a Highly Convective Flow. *Appl. Phys. Lett.* **16**, 214–217.

Bulthius, K. (1973). Laser Power and Vibrational Energy Transfer in CO_2 Lasers. *J. Chem. Phys.* **58**, 5786–5794.

Buonadonna, V. R., and Christiansen, W. H. (1973). Gain Measurements of High Temperature CO_2 Laser Mixtures in a Shock Tube Driven Flow. *Recent Dev. Shock Tube Res.* Stanford Univ. Press, Stanford, California, 174–183.

Christiansen, W. H., and Tsongas, G. A. (1971). Gain Kinetics of CO_2 Gasdynamic Laser Mixtures at High Pressure. *Phys. Fluids* **14**, 2611–2619.

Chroshko, V. N., Soloukhin, R. I., and Wolanski, P. (1972). Population Inversion by Mixing in a Shock Tube Flow. *Opt. Commun.* **6**, 275–277.

Chroshko, V. N., Soloukhin, R. I., and Wolanski, P. (1973). Population Inversion by Mixing in a Shock Tube Flow. *Recent Dev. Shock Tube Res.*, Stanford Univ. Press, Stanford, California, 167–172.

Clark, P. O. (1972). Design Considerations for High Power Laser Cavities. AIAA Paper No. 72–708.

Clarke, J. F., and McChesney, M. (1964). *The Dynamics of Real Gases.* Butterworth, London.

Courant, R., Friedrichs, K. O., and Levy, H. (1928). Ueber die Differenzengleichungen der Mathematischen Physik. *Math. Ann.* **100**, 32.

Davidson, N. (1962). *Statistical Mechanics.* McGraw-Hill, New York.

De Temple, T. A., Suhre, D. R., and Coleman, P. D. (1973). Relaxation Rates of Lower Laser Levels in CO_2. *Appl. Phys. Lett.* **22**, 349–350.

Director, M. N. (1973). Aerodynamic Parameters Affecting Practical Gas Dynamic Laser Design. AIAA Paper No. 73–626.

Fisher, E. R., and Smith, G. K. (1970). Vibrational Relaxation by Metal Atoms. *Chem. Phys. Lett.* **6**, 438–440.

Gabai, A., Rokni, M., Greenfield, E., Dothan-Deutsch, F., and Yatsiv, S. (1972). CO_2 Gasdynamic Laser by Detonation of a Solid Explosive. Presented at the VII Int. Quantum Electron. Conf., Montreal.

Gembarzhevskiy, G. V., Generalov, N. A., Kozlov, G. I., and Roytenburg, D. I. (1972). Amplification Factor of Light in a CO_2, N_2, He Mixture as It Expands in a Supersonic Nozzle. *Zh. Eksp. Teor. Fiz.* **62**, 844–847.

Gerry, E. T. (1970). Gasdynamic Lasers. *IEEE Spectrum* **7**, 51–58.

Gerry, E. T., and Leonard, D. A. (1966). Measurements of 10.6 μ CO_2 Laser Transition Probability and Optical Broadening Cross Sections. *Appl. Phys. Lett.* **8**, 227–229.

Glowacki, W. J., and Anderson, J. D., Jr. (1971). A Computer Program for CO_2–N_2–H_2O Gasdynamic Laser Gain and Maximum Available Power. NOLTR 71–210. Naval Ordnance Lab., White Oak, Maryland.

Greenberg, R. A., Schneiderman, A. M., Ahouse, D. R., and Parmentier, E. M. (1970). Rapid Expansion Nozzles for Gas Dynamic Lasers. AVCO Res. Lab. AMP 314.

Hall, J. G., and Treanor, C. E. (1967). Nonequilibrium Effects in Supersonic-Nozzle Flows. AGARD-ograph No. 124.

Hertzberg, A., Johnston, E. W., and Ahlstrom, H. G. (1972). Photon Generators and Engines for Laser Power Transmission. *AIAA J.* **10**, 394–400.

Hoffman, A. L., and Jones, T. G. (1972). Geometrical Methods for Improving the Optical Quality of Gasdynamic Lasers. AIAA Paper No. 72–217.

Hoffman, A. L., and Vlases, G. C. (1972). A Simplified Model for Predicting Gain, Saturation, and Pulse Length for Gas Dynamic Lasers. *IEEE Quantum Electron.* **QE-8**, 46–53.

Howgate, D. W., Roberts, T. G., and Barr, T. A. (1972). Numerical Calculation of the Arc-Driven Supersonic Laser Operating in the Gas Dynamic Mode. *J. Appl. Phys.* **43,** 2799–2804.

Hurle, I. R., and Hertzberg, A. (1965). Electronic Population Inversions by Fluid–Mechanical Techniques. *Phys. Fluids* **8,** 1601–1607.

Kantrowitz, A. R. (1946). Heat Capacity Lag in Gas Dynamics. *J. Chem. Phys.* **14,** 150–164.

Klosterman, E. L., and Hoffman, A. L. (1973). A High Pressure Shock Tube Driven Gasdynamic Laser. *Recent Dev. Shock Tube Res.* Stanford Univ. Press, Stanford, California, 156–166.

Kogelnik, H., and Li, T. (1966). Laser Beams and Resonators. *Appl. Opt.* **5,** 1550–1567.

Kuehn, D. M., and Monson, D. J. (1970). Experiments with a CO_2 Gasdynamic Laser. *Appl. Phys. Lett.* **16,** 48–50.

Lee, G. (1974). Quasi-One-Dimensional Solution for the Power of CO_2 Gasdynamic Lasers. *Phys. Fluids* **17,** 644–649.

Lee, G., and Gowen, F. E. (1971). Gain of CO_2 Gasdynamic Lasers. *Appl. Phys. Lett.* **18,** 237–239.

Lee, G., Gowen, F. E., and Hagen, J. R. (1972). Gain and Power of CO_2 Gasdynamic Lasers. *AIAA J.* **10,** 65–71.

Lengyel, B. A. (1971). *Lasers*, 2nd ed. Wiley (Interscience), New York.

Liepmann, H. W., and Roshko, A. (1957). *Elements of Gasdynamics.* Wiley, New York.

MacCormack, R. W. (1969). The Effect of Viscosity in Hypervelocity Impact Cratering. AIAA Paper No. 69–354.

MacDonald, J. R. (1970). Rate Coefficients for Vibrational Energy Transfer in Rapid Expansions of Carbon Dioxide–Nitrogen Mixtures. SUIPR Rep. No. 394, Inst. Plasma Res., Stanford Univ., Stanford, California.

Madden, M. T., Anderson, J. D., Jr., and Piper, C. H. (1970). Equilibrium Normal Shock Properties for Vibrationally Excited CO_2–N_2–He Gas Mixtures. NOLTR 70–103. Naval Ordnance Lab., White Oak, Maryland.

McKenzie, R. L. (1972). Diatomic Gasdynamic Lasers. *Phys. Fluids* **15,** 2163–2173.

McLeary, R. (1972). Calculation of Gain and Power Output for a Gas Dynamic Laser. *IEEE J. Quantum Electron.* **QE-8,** 716–718.

Meinzer, R. A. (1972). Experimental Gasdynamic Laser Studies. *AIAA J.* **10,** 388–393.

Milewski, J., Brunne, M., Stanco, J., Zielinski, A., Irczuk, M., and Kusmierek, J. (1972). CW Gasdynamic Thermally Excited and Selectively Pumped CO_2–N_2 Mixing Laser. *Bull. Acad. Pol. Sci.* **20,** 313–319.

Monsler, M. J., and Greenberg, R. A. (1971). The Effects of Boundary Layers on the Gain of a Gasdynamic Laser. AIAA Paper 71–24.

Munjee, S. A. (1970). An Analysis of Population Inversion in the Supersonic Expansion of CO_2 Laser Mixtures. MS Thesis, Dept. of Mechanical Engineering, Univ. of Washington.

Munjee, S. A. (1972). Numerical Analysis of a Gasdynamic Laser Mixture. *Phys. Fluids* **15,** 506–508.

Murray, E. R., Jr. (1974). Vibrational Nonequilibrium in Carbon Dioxide Electric Discharge Lasers. SUIPR Rep. No. 562, Inst. Plasma Res., Stanford Univ., Stanford, California.

Murty, S. S. R. (1974). Rapid Estimation of the Performance Characteristics of CO_2 Gasdynamic Lasers. AIAA Paper No. 74–226.

Pallay, B. G., and Zovko, C. T. (1973). Fuels, Oxidizers and Gas Generators for Gas Dynamic Lasers. AIAA Paper No. 73–1233.

Parmentier, E. M. (1972). Supersonic Flow Aerodynamic Windows for High Power Lasers. AIAA Paper No. 72–710.

Patel, C. K. N. (1968). High Power Carbon Dioxide Lasers. *Sci. Am.* **219,** 22–33.

Rigrod, W. W. (1965). Saturation Effects in High-Gain Lasers. *Appl. Phys.* **36,** 2487–2490.

Rosser, W. A., Jr., Hoag, E., and Gerry, E. T. (1972). Relaxation of Excess Populations in the Lower Laser Level CO_2 (100). *J. Chem. Phys.* **57,** 4153–4164.

Royle, J. K., Bowling, A. G., and Lukasiewicz, J. (1947). Calibration of Two-Dimensional and Conical Supersonic Multi-Nozzles. RAE Rep. AERO 2221. R. Aeronaut. Establishment, England.

Russell, D. A. (1974). Fluid Mechanics of High Power Grid Nozzle Lasers. AIAA Paper No. 74–223.

Sato, K., and Sekiguchi, T. (1973). Dependence of the Output Power of CO_2 Gas Dynamic Laser on the Distance from Nozzle Throat. *J. Phys. Soc. Jpn.* **35,** 630.

Schwartz, R. N., Slawsky, Z. I., and Herzfeld, K. F. (1952). Calculation of Vibrational Relaxation Times in Gases. *J. Chem. Phys.* **20,** 1591–1599.

Shapiro, A. H. (1953). *The Dynamics and Thermodynamics of Compressible Fluid Flow.* Ronald Press, New York.

Sharma, R. D. (1971). Vibrational Relaxation of CO_2 by H_2O. *J. Chem. Phys.* **54,** 810–811.

Siegman, A. E. (1971). *An Introduction to Lasers and Masers.* McGraw-Hill, New York.

Simons, G. A. (1972). The Effect of Boundary Layers on GDL Medium Homogeniety. AIAA Paper No. 72–709.

Sutton, G. W. (1969). Effect of Turbulent Fluctuations in an Optically Active Fluid Medium. *AIAA J.* **7,** 1737–1743.

Taran, J. P. E., Charpenel, M., and Borghi, R. (1973). Investigation of a Mixing CO_2 GDL. AIAA Paper No. 73–622.

Taylor, R. L., and Bitterman, S. (1967). Survey of Vibrational Relaxation Data for Processes Important in the CO_2–N_2 Laser System. Avco Everett Res. Rep. 282.

Taylor, R. L., and Bitterman, S. (1969). Survey of Vibrational Relaxation Data for Processes Important in the CO_2–N_2 Laser System. *Rev. Mod. Phys.* **41,** 26–47.

Teare, J. D., Taylor, R. L., and von Rosenberg, C. W. (1970). Observations of Vibration–Vibration Energy Pumping Between Diatomic Molecules. *Nature* **225,** 240–243.

Tennant, R., Vargas, R., and Hadley, S. (1974). Effects of Gaseous Contaminants on Gasdynamic Laser Performance. AIAA Paper No. 74–178.

Treanor, C. E., Rich, J. W., and Rehm, R. G. (1968). Vibrational Relaxation of Anharmonic Oscillators with Exchange-Dominated Collisions. *J. Chem. Phys.* **48,** 1798–1807.

Tulip, J., and Sequin, H. (1971). Explosion-Pumped Gas Dynamic CO_2 Laser. *Appl. Phys. Lett.* **19,** 263–265.

Vamos, J. S. (1974). Small-Signal Gain Measurements in a High-Ratio Nozzle Shock Tunnel GDL. AIAA Paper No. 74–177.

Vincenti, W. G., and Kruger, C. H. (1965). *Introduction to Physical Gas Dynamics.* Wiley, New York.

Wagner, J. L. (1971). A Cold Flow Field Experimental Study Associated with a Two-Dimensional Multiple Nozzle. NOLTR 71–78. Naval Ordnance Lab., White Oak, Maryland.

Warren, W. R. (1959). Determination of Air Stagnation Properties in High-Enthalpy Test Facility. *J. Aeronaut. Sci.* **26,** 835–836.

Winkler, E. M., Humphrey, R. L., and Koenig, J. A. (1970). The NOL Four-Ring Three-Phase AC Arc Heater (MKIV). NOLTR 70–12. Naval Ordnance Lab., White Oak, Maryland.

Yatsiv, S., Greenfield, E., Dothan–Deutsch, F., Chuchem, D., and Bin–Nun, E. (1971). Pulsed CO_2 Gasdynamic Laser. *Appl. Phys. Lett.* **19,** 65–68.

Index

O

P

R

S

T

A 6
B 7
C 8
D 9
E 0
F 1
G 2
H 3
I 4
J 5